# Praise for *Close to OM*

"Andrea's combination of a challenging class and a great sense of humor are unique, intelligent, and always leave me feeling better when I leave than when I arrived. She is an amazing teacher, and I love her class."—Heather Graham

"Reading through *Close to OM* is a light and airy foray into yoga. Andrea Marcum presents yoga as a serious but fun and doable practice, with lots of good tips—both on and off the mat. Her delightful stories and metaphors make it easy to understand why we might want to incorporate yoga into our daily lives for a more peaceful, happy, and healthy existence."
—Beryl Bender Birch, bestselling author of *Power Yoga* and director/founder of The Hard & The Soft Yoga Institute

"Ten years ago, Andrea introduced me to yoga and she has been my teacher ever since. *Close to OM* is like having a little Andrea inside your head! She writes the way she teaches—with honesty, humor, and inspiration."—Noah Baumbach, filmmaker/director

"At our executive retreat, Andrea convinced even the most skeptical on our team that mindfulness and yoga are exciting tools to improve our quality of life and job performance. Her approachable style allowed everyone to feel comfortable and made the session a great success."—Michael Edelstein, president, NBCUniversal International Television Production

"Andrea Marcum is vitality and grace personified. To meet her is to know her. She is truly fully expressed and the embodiment of love in every moment—inspiring you to laugh a little louder and love a little harder. As you flow through the pages of *Close to OM*, you feel as if she is alongside you personally, guiding you throughout the process. Andrea is a brilliant teacher, committed to being of service to others, and a forever student—contagiously curious about the world. *Close to OM* will invite you inside Andrea's knowledge, curiosity, and heart—you'll leave with a renewed sense of inquisitiveness, inspiration, and guidance."
—Sarah Harvison, lululemon Global Yoga Ambassador Program Manager

"In *Close to OM*, Andrea's vulnerable, accessible honesty invites you onto the path. She's an expert at guiding you to embrace your unique potential and at making you feel she's right there with you as you do."—Liz Hernandez, host, *Access Hollywood*

"In *Close to OM*, Andrea takes us down a path that reinforces why yoga is so important to our often chaotic lives. I am grateful to have her as a steadfast and inspiring guide on my own journey."—Shannon Furman, producer, NFL Network

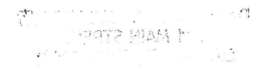

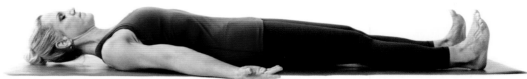

# STRETCHING YOGA FROM

# Close *to* OM

## YOUR MAT TO YOUR LIFE

## Andrea Marcum

ST. MARTIN'S GRIFFIN ✦ NEW YORK

www.stmartins.com

Book design by Richard Oriolo

PHOTO CREDITS:
Janie Robertson, p. 9, 12, 39, 117, 129, 160; Kiki Elrod, p. 10; Guy Shalem, p. 20, 64; Mirey Attalah, p. 122; Andrea Marcum, p. 169, 180; Fluid Frame, p. 182; All other photos and cover courtesy of Patricia Pena

Illustrations by Andrea Marcum

The Library of Congress Cataloging-in-Publication Data is available upon request.

ISBN 978-1-250-12759-4 (trade paperback)
ISBN 978-1-250-12760-0 (ebook)

Our books may be purchased in bulk for promotional, educational, or business use. Please contact your local bookseller or the Macmillan Corporate and Premium Sales Department at 1-800-221-7945, extension 5442, or by email at MacmillanSpecialMarkets@macmillan.com.

FIRST EDITION: January 2018

10 9 8 7 6 5 4 3 2 1

For all of my teachers

ॐ

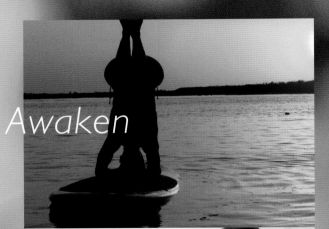

Awaken

Transform

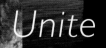

Unite

# CONTENTS

**I HAD MY FIRST RUN-IN** with yoga in the '70s. I can't remember if it was Lilias Folan on TV or if I started with my workbooks at home, but somehow I got turned on to yoga at fifteen years old. And then I got off onto my whole drugs-wild-lifestyle and drifted away from yoga. I moved to LA in 1990 and started taking flow classes with people like Bryan Kest and Seane Corn. Then, because I had no idea what to do with my life, Grace Slick told me, "You've got really strong legs, you dig this yoga stuff, try that. " And she gave me money to go to White Lotus and do my first teacher training.

Not long after White Lotus, I was at 24-Hour Fitness, the teacher didn't show up, and the two other people in the room said, "Why don't you teach the class?" Despite my training I really had no clue what I was doing. But I did know that when we practice we come in with such mishigas, tumult, stuff from the world, our worries, anxieties. Then we practice, and all of a sudden something shifts. We get up out of savasana and think,

"Wow, I feel a lot more peaceful and calm—I've got a different perspective on life."

Yoga has seen me through treatments for hepatitis C from my intravenous drug use in the '70s and '80s. And it has kept me grounded and healthy enough to be celebrating thirty-two years of being clean and sober as I write this. My years of teaching have made me aware that underneath every "normal-looking" person there's divorce, illness, fear, mental instability, financial issues. We're all going through so much. That's why Andrea Marcum's book *Close to OM: Stretching Yoga from Your Mat to Your Life* is so important. Andrea shows us that yoga doesn't mean you have to do gymnastics. In fact, the real transformation comes out of the stillness. With her unique voice she guides us out from under where we're Stuckat (to use her word) and toward a better understanding of what brings purpose and meaning to our lives.

I met Andrea many years ago in my classroom in Los Angeles. Even back then, she had a fire about her. She was an intense student who'd show up pretty much every day to my flow classes wearing her baggy black Thai-style pants looking ready for jujitsu. Andrea's passionate about learning. As I've watched her evolve from student to teacher, she's stayed on the path of being a seeker—questioning and truly integrating what she's learning into what she feels is real. Andrea isn't afraid to take risks. Whether that's opening a studio in LA, organizing her own retreats, or writing—she puts it all out there, travels, grows, and is committed to really looking at the integrity behind what she's doing.

*Close to OM* is accessible for newer students while it resonates with those of us who have been taking or even teaching yoga for years.

Andrea's combination of relatable stories, down-to-earth philosophy mixed with clear alignment points, and straightforward meditation invites us all into a conversation that's as fun as it is serious. She manages to make us laugh as we learn about ourselves, about yoga, and about life.

—Vinnie Marino

# Introduction

**I WAS IN THE SIXTH GRADE** when I discovered gymnastics. One typically foggy afternoon, my mom dropped my friend Addie and me off at the Santa Cruz Gymnastics Center. Located in Northern California, Santa Cruz is part college town, part beach town. The UC Santa Cruz campus stares down at the Beach Boardwalk and Fisherman's Wharf from stunning redwood forest hills. I grew up there, when middle-aged mothers surfed Steamer's Lane and men with shoulder-length beards in "No Nukes" T-shirts and vintage VW buses were at nearly every intersection. *Organic, wheatgrass juice,* and *soy milk* were commonplace vernacular long before they hit the mainstream.

The Santa Cruz Gymnastics Center was the first legitimate competitive gymnastics program in the county. It was there that Steve, our raw-garlic-clove-consuming, Robert Bly–worshipping teacher, introduced Addie and me to tumbling, balance beam, uneven parallel bars, and vaulting horse. In the years to come, gymnastics would be my blessing and my curse.

I spent endless hours smelling the sprouted wheat bread baking at the Staff of Life Natural Food Market next door while I tore the calluses on my parallel-bar hands and destroyed my ankles with the full twisting layouts in my floor routine—all in the hopes that Steve would decide during one of his drum circles to put me on the competitive squad. Little did I know finding my way onto the team would introduce me to an albatross I would spend decades attempting to shake.

The pressures of body image were mounting. Being a teenager sucks, and being a gymnast while you're a teenager is even worse. Addie was told she was too thin and not strong enough. I'd been put on diet after diet to try to get the fat girl slim. In an average-girl lineup, I wouldn't have stood out as corpulent. But by gymnastic standards, I was a lard-ass, and they weren't afraid to let me know it.

There was no room for self-acceptance in the competitive gymnast agenda, which queued me up for years rife with self-loathing (even beyond my adolescence). All those hours in the gym had left me stocky, muscle-bound, and flat-chested. We were expected to be ballerina thin and yet to perform physical feats that required us to be strong like little boys. Our coaching was like being handed *Men's Fitness* when what we really needed was *Are You There God? It's Me, Margaret*. It made for a schizophrenic coming-of-age, one that tried desperately to put puberty on pause. I competed for four years, starting in proficiency Class Three and moving up to Class Two. My weight yo-yoed up and down, but somehow never down enough for Class One.

The preoccupation with stick-thin slenderness and humiliating weigh-ins wasn't the only blow to my self-image. I was sporting a very unfortunate Dorothy Hamill haircut, made worse by an abundance of cowlicks. Silver braces covered my buck teeth like train tracks struggling to cinch the gaping abyss between the front two. Because I refused to wear the painful nightly neck gear that had been assigned, any actual correction would be a long time coming.

It also didn't help that I was "Andy."

One summer when my mother, my brothers, and I were in New York City for a visit, I wandered into the ladies' room in Central Park. "Oh, the little boys' room is around the corner," a startled East Coast accent belted in my direction. When I noticed everyone looking at me I froze. A flash of bright red across my mistaken-for-male face . . . How could I defend my female-ness? If only my mother had let me get my ears pierced the way I'd been begging her—surely that would have spared me (as it does androgynous Italian and Latin American baby girls everywhere) the humiliation of being called "he." Devastated, I caved, ran outside, and burst into tears.

Without missing a beat, my mother took me by the hand and stormed back in. "This is my daughter and she is *beautiful*," she thundered. I was completely embarrassed, but it was the first time she'd ever said that about me. From that point on, my mother frequently cited Liv Ullmann's ascent from ugly duckling to celebrated beauty and Ingmar Bergman muse. This never made sense to me. Liv was stunning Norwegian fairness from day one. But Gwen Marcum's version of Liv's story became my Holy Grail.

Increasingly, the gorilla suit covering my lack of self-esteem was my weight, a suit I wore out of the gym and into the world. The physiological map for weight loss is pretty straightforward: burn more calories than you take in. It's an annoyingly elementary fact. The psychology of weight loss can be a bit murkier . . .

Covert eating began as a sporadic, secret means of comfort during my gymnastics days, and then grew into a full-blown adversarial relationship with food. Sure, it would squelch my frustrations temporarily, but then binger's remorse took hold. Food was in turn my best friend, then my worst enemy, and I had no idea how to get off the gorge-purge Ferris wheel.

In college, when I tried out for the production of *A Chorus Line*, there were a lot of whispers behind the audition table. "Do you think you look like a Broadway dancer?" the director asked me in front of everyone. And I mean *everyone*. The nearly two hundred people auditioning were seated in the red velvet seats of the Bovard Auditorium, staring at me. The choreographer, whose class I took regularly, shook her head in shame next to him. "Sweetheart, you're just too heavy to be believable." I wanted to die, or at the very least throw up. Actually, one of the dancers who made it into the show told me to try using laxatives. "That's what all us dancers do." Suffice to say it was ineffective and short lived . . . and I went up a pant size by semester's end.

After college I was a singer-songwriter/miserable waitress in LA for a few too many years at Angeli Caffe, a wonderful little Italian café on Melrose. Angeli had *the* best round loaves of bread, hot from the pizza oven. Unlike the sprouted wheat bread at Staff of Life, far too many of these Angeli loaves made their way home with me. I never ate them in front of people. Instead I stashed them away for later. If no one saw me consuming, I thought, then it didn't count.

My life became days of starvation filled with spin classes, circuit training, "cardio funk," and "step and pump." After all, being in the gym was what I knew. Then I would collapse into a lonely vat of salt, sugar, and fat, with so little food value it wasn't allowed to make eye contact with the nutrition pyramid and so many calories that not even an uninterrupted twenty-four hours on the elliptical would burn them all.

In no way did I believe what my mother had blurted out to strangers in that Central Park restroom. I was a long way from feeling beautiful like Liv.

There was one huge positive I took away from my early gymnastics days: the incredible discipline I learned at a young age. I was tubby, but determined and willing to log the hours no matter what anyone said. Like my albatross, determination also followed me out of the gym and into my life. The problem was, my discipline didn't allow for any joy. Nothing was ever enough.

It was the introduction of downward facing dog to my strong will that eventually led me toward the path of self-acceptance.

Oh, I know how precious it sounds for me to say that yoga changed my life. So let's just get that part out in the open.

It did.

And I've watched it change other people's lives, too. But let's also not fool ourselves. Transformation isn't instant, it isn't particularly cute, and it isn't easy. It *is* insightful, pretty funny at times, and incredibly rewarding. "Less is more" was to me an annoying cliché one might find in a fortune cookie. But the stillness and quiet of my first down dog was so loud and unnerving it refused to be denied. No machines, no spin shoes or booming sound system.

Just me.

My relationship with my weight was the first thing yoga helped me begin to untangle. It became a portal for me to peer through so I could take a look at the big ship. For the first time in my life, I was learning how to log off and sit with things instead of filling everything (including myself) up. My yoga practice was like a visit to the therapist: contemplative, confronting, and fundamentally calming. I'd made other physical endeavors extreme and punishing, which only fed my feeding cycle. There's actually a scientific explanation for this. The persistent stress my Ferris wheel lifestyle was creating had my adrenals pumping hormones like cortisol into my system rapid-fire. Cortisol is linked to weight gain, not only because it shuts down digestion but because it also makes us crave the high-sugar, high-carbohydrate foods we refer to as "comfort foods."

Yoga nurtured a part of me I hadn't yet met. Learning to be nonreactive on my mat gave me insight into reactive behavior off my mat. Realizing that I was unconsciously biting my lip while I practiced became a gateway to addressing the other things I was biting into that I didn't need.

One of the central texts in yoga philosophy is Patanjali's *Yoga Sutras*. It's a string of aphorisms considered to be the most complete and organized definition of the discipline. Verse 2:46 speaks of *sthira sukham asanum*, which translates as a steady, easeful pose. If applied to a higher sense of self-realization, it becomes the missing piece essential to all personal transformation. Yes, I had to be solid and steady in my commitment, but I also needed to learn how to enjoy and find ease. I needed to be flexible in the ways that mattered most. As I did, it became less about being fat or thin, and more about being well nourished in all respects.

I started feeling deserving, and because of that I wanted to immerse myself, and my life, in habits that felt good. Slowly I was learning to make things manageable, and lo and behold they became enjoyable, too. I turned off the TV and read *The Essential Rumi*, *Siddhartha*, Rilke's *Letters to a Young Poet*, *Bird by Bird*, and *The Four Agreements*, not *People* magazine . . . well, not as often. I visited the Erewhon natural foods market salad bar far more frequently than the Ralph's ice cream aisle or the corner store's chip section. I wore colors other than black and allowed myself cute fitted tops (the bottoms would take a few more years of convincing—they were a bigger issue, and yes, I mean that in every way). I was enriched and, as a result, satiated. As I became more comfortable being *with* myself, I became more comfortable *being* myself.

Two years after my first down dog I signed up for a teacher training, and I've now been teaching for about seventeen years. Though I'd have voted myself Least Likely to Be an

Entrepreneur, I opened U Studio Yoga in Los Angeles in 2006 and ran it for nine years. Then yoga stretched me out into the world to teach and lead retreats, which made it difficult to run an independent studio on my own, so in April 2015, I closed U Studio.

As grateful as I am to travel the globe, I'm even more thankful that yoga has helped me travel far from my nothing's ever enough/miserable waitress days. My practice, both postural and philosophical, has guided me to develop the guided journey you're about to discover in these pages. Through my personal exploration I've learned to stand in what I call my Val-you and Truth, and I've been able to S.T.O.P. punitive patterns and S.T.A.R.T. again in ways that have led me toward love—first for myself and then in the form of my wonderful husband, Dom, and the most amazing community of like-minded practitioners. I'm thrilled to share these principles with you and invite you with open arms into the OM collective.

Maybe, like me, you too have found yoga at your gym or are interested in it as a form of exercise. The physical incentive is a great place to start. B. K. S. Iyengar (the father of the Iyengar style of yoga) said, "Penetration of the mind is our goal, but in the beginning there is no substitute for sweat." People ask me all the time if my class is hard enough to be a workout. Will it give them ripped abs, a swimsuit model's butt, and Madonna's arms? Make them look ten years younger? Living in LA, it's as if everybody's desperate to be camera-ready all the time even if they aren't actually going to be in front of a camera. So you'd assume my class reviews and testimonials would be all butt cheeks, biceps, and six-packs, right?

But when you ask my students, it's not physical accomplishment they point to when they talk about how our yoga together has transformed their lives. It's something more far-reaching. For example, when he introduced me to a group of his executives that I was teaching in the English countryside, the president of NBCUniversal International said, "Andrea showed me that how you do your yoga is how you do your life."

And that's what *Close to OM* is going to do for you.

It is your personal guide to how to do your yoga to create the life you want. It reveals yoga as a tool to get beneath what's superficial and awaken to who you really are—not who you purport yourself to be on your LinkedIn or online-dating profile, but your sincere, authentic essence—body, mind, and spirit. When you embrace who you really are you become crystal clear about what matters, what gives you purpose, and how to fully inhabit your best life. In these pages I offer some of the practices and exercises I've found most helpful both for myself and for my students. You will use poses as gateways to dig deep into the "head, hands, and heart" of your unique psychology. You are going to integrate yoga into your life as a means to find your way to your full, unique potential, and yoga's yoke of body, mind, and spiritual teachings is going to get you there both on and off your mat.

*Close to OM* is not a catalog of yoga styles to help you pick a certain type of class or an encyclopedia of all the poses ever invented. Together, you and I will navigate how to use your yoga to stretch past where you're feeling limited both in your practice and out in the world. Whether you consider yourself a beginner or super advanced, *Close to OM* is a straightforward roadmap that leads you beyond those things—physical, mental, and spiritual—that are keeping you from doing and being what you want. It's a system that gets you past your fear, self-sabotage, limiting beliefs, and other inhibiting behaviors and replaces them with creativity, productivity, contentment, and well-being.

Believe me, I understand that working our muscles feels immediate and palpable. Almost instantly we feel like we are inviting progress in some way. I also know that if we're going to truly liberate ourselves, focusing only on our bodies will not be enough. And I completely appreciate that concepts like philosophy and psychology can initially seem heady, esoteric, and irrelevant. Without the right translator they feel like a college elective you know you should take but can't see any use for in your real life. I'm not delivering a doctoral dissertation or claiming to have invented yoga. Nor am I going to hand you ethereal hocus-pocus, try to turn you into someone you aren't, or overwhelm you with an impossible game plan. In fact, I think you'll find my writing and instruction is designed more for the everyperson than it is for those select few who can effortlessly tie their bodies into a bow and appear always to have their shit together.

Our odyssey is more like an archeological dig to discover the hidden treasures that already exist within you but have become buried and lost underneath obstacles you might not yet be able to see. Our core work will run much deeper than simply sculpting our bodies. We are going to empower ourselves to shape our own inspired reality. Together we will use the physical immediacy of postures and the transformational tools yoga offers, and you too will discover that "how you do your yoga is how you do your life."

And if you end up sporting a stronger set of abs, too, well that's no crime, is it?

In this book, you and I will be going on a journey to learn about how you can use yoga to change your life—body, mind, and spirit. There's a wonderfully interactive feeling to our journey. It's a bit like heading off on a retreat together, one that requires no airline ticket or baggage fee, one that's accessible from anywhere at any time. At the end of this book, you will know a lot more about yoga and its poses, but you'll also know more about you: who you are, what you want, and how to get there—on and off your mat. Our time together is organized into three sections:

> You first *awaken* to the present moment, creating enough space in your physical body and in your cluttered mind to begin again and establish a fresh new canvas for change.
>
> You then *transform*, integrating physical postures with cognitive and emotional discovery—synthesizing long respected traditions with modern-day reality and your own body's individual needs. Your poses are conduits to better understand what you're feeling—first in your hamstrings and then in your heart. As you recognize what you're feeling, you comprehend better what you're thinking, the choices you're making, and whether your actions are leading you toward what you want or simply reinforcing cycles of what you don't.
>
> Lastly, we *unite* with compassion, intuition, integrity, and a connection to your highest self and to the world around you. Ultimately alignment is more than just whether or not your knee is lined up with your pinky toe; it is aligning with a greater good.

Though our journey is divided into *awaken, transform,* and *unite,* ultimately these three parts intermingle as an organic whole just like yoga's union of body, mind, and spirit. Yoga is ever-deepening and lifelong, and you can return to any section of this book to begin again and again. **Close to OM** is not a destination outside of yourself that you're trying to get to. It is a path to the rich, extraordinary wisdom within.

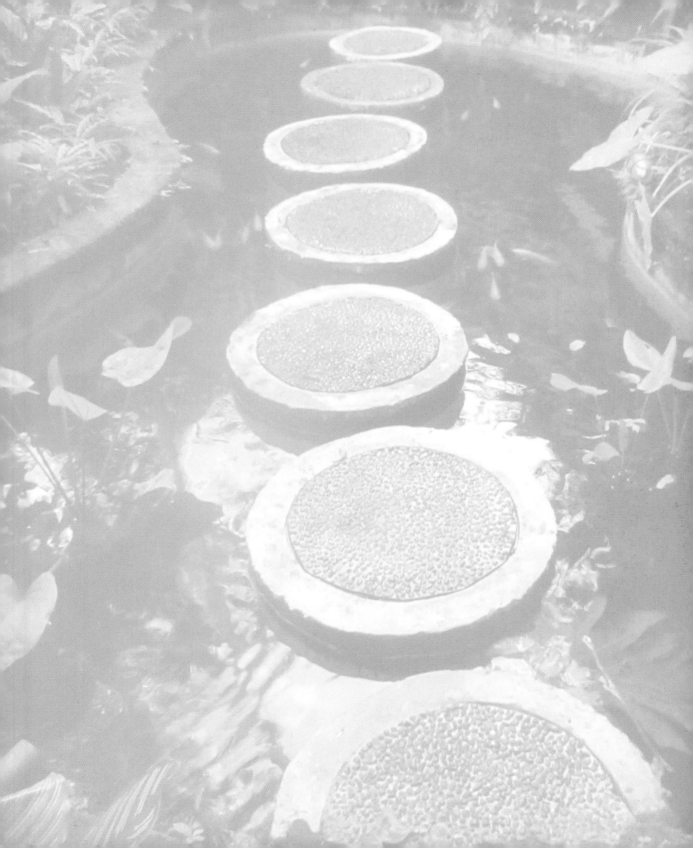

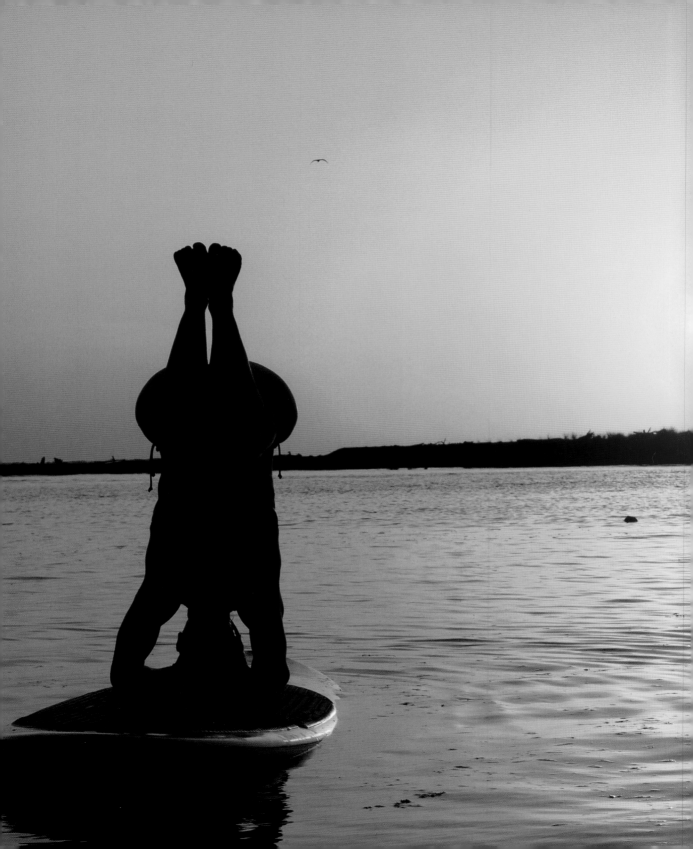

# PART I

# AWAKEN

In this section you *awaken*. **Awakening is the first step in a shift toward positive change. You S.T.O.P. to S.T.A.R.T.—awakening to who and where you really are. You land in your breath and in the present moment, discover the inspiration of your beginner's mind, and create an internal and external environment conducive to transformation.**

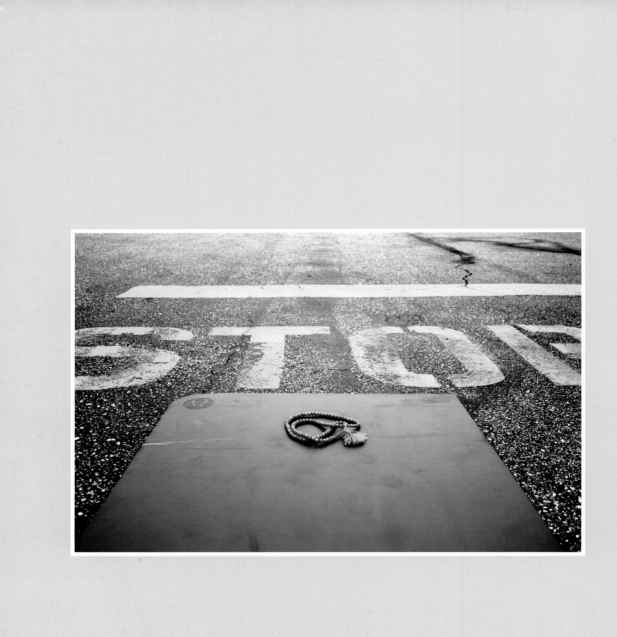

# S.T.O.P. to S.T.A.R.T.

*When you stop to take a flower*
*in your hand and really look at it,*
*it's your world for that moment.*

—GEORGIA O'KEEFFE

**In this chapter you *awaken* to the fact that you must stop in order to start.**

You most likely know savasana (or corpse pose) as that moment at the end of a yoga practice when you stop and lie down. I'm going to tell you savasana is the beginning.

Savasana is the perfect place for us to S.T.O.P. so that we can S.T.A.R.T.

**S.** **Stop** moving, fixing, fidgeting, thinking about the past, or anticipating the future.

**T.** **Take one breath at a time.**

**O.** **Observe.** Is your jaw tight? Does something itch? Are you tapping your fingers or fidgety in your feet? What are you feeling? Thinking? Hearing? Just notice.

**P.** **Pause before proceeding.** Resist the temptation to jump ahead and move on. Let yourself simply be here observing for a moment.

Then . . .

**S.** **Start to make space.** Space is where possibility lives. Feel the capacity to create space in your body, mind, and breath. Start with the space between your fingers and toes, between your shoulders and your ears, and between your inhales and exhales.

**T.** **Turn down the volume.** Feel as though you have your hand on the volume knob of negative chatter, distractions, and excuses, and start to turn the volume down.

**A.** **Accept and acknowledge.** Accept where you are right now and start to acknowledge room for expansion and improvement without finding fault.

**R.** **Renew.** Let spacious, quiet acceptance facilitate your new start.

**T.** **Take thoughtful action.**

Only then can we *awaken*. Awakening is the first step in a shift toward positive change. In our body and mind we're like those snow globes you shake and fill with chaotic, blinding snow until we stop, breathe, and let the snow of our agitated bodies and overstimulated minds subside—allowing us to awaken to the landscape within.

When we S.T.O.P. we can let go of our elusive quest for worldly solutions to our unhappiness, and S.T.A.R.T. to allow a quieter, more genuine joy to come to the surface. It's a pause for us to "be" instead of perpetuating the constant and tumultuous "doing" our lives can be reduced to. The anticipation of knowing we have to rush to reach our destination, meet our deadline, or live up to imposed expectations can be a real buzz kill, making it nearly impossible to sit still. But if we don't S.T.O.P. the madness, how can any of us shift our internal climate from turbulent to temperate?

As a yoga teacher, I've watched thousands of agitated bodies, tapping hands and feet, darting eyes, and clearly spinning minds struggle to stay where they are until I set them free. Restlessness can be very convincing. In my classes I have some serial savasana duckers, those who skip it and leave early every time. As a student even I have had those times where I've spent almost the entire class planning my escape, plotting the moment when I could slip out unnoticed and hurl myself back into the comfort of the insanity outside. Only to be reassured that like an unfinished conversation, leaving midstream is never satisfying.

So how do we access this subtle landscape that leads us ultimately to more freedom, calm, and possibility? Just as we do with athletic poses like arm-balances and backbends, we need to allow ourselves to discover in increments. I believe it's important to start by breaking things into manageable bits. I'm not asking you to sign a contract for twenty-minute headstands, days of solemn silence, and zero signs of fun—just bite-size, easily digested practices you can do consistently before you decide whether you're going to the gym or if you should reach for the remote, sautéing or steaming your broccoli, and if you should return those shoes you bought.

In my classroom, before we begin, the first thing we do is S.T.O.P. so that we can S.T.A.R.T. We climb onto our mats and into a child's pose or comfortable seat to pause and let both ourselves and the room settle. Though physically we may not be sprawled out on the floor in the typical savasana position, mentally and emotionally we are taking a savasana of sorts. As you begin your journey **Close to OM** you must do the same, S.T.O.P. to S.T.A.R.T.—create a conscious savasana time-out so you can tune in.

B. K. S. Iyengar likens savasana to a snake shedding its dead skin to reveal the vibrant colors of newness beneath. Our S.T.O.P. to S.T.A.R.T. savasana allows us to let go of what is not needed so we can blossom anew.

## ON YOUR MAT

In this book we're going to do a number of exercises together that involve marinating in the assignment for a certain amount of time. First, you'll read through the instruction, then you'll use any method of time-keeping that works for you: your phone, a setting on your watch, a good old fashioned cooking timer, or you can use @OM in the dropdown menu at www.closetoOM.com. There you'll find audio guidance for the exercise you've just read, and the timing is all taken care of for you.

Within these pages, you and I may find ourselves doing the same yoga pose, but we will never have exactly the same experience while we're in it. Some of us are inspired to expedite the end zone, while others enjoy a slower, more methodical strategy. Personally, I've come back to this material over and over again, year after year—sometimes moving through things linearly and often revisiting and lingering in specific chapters and principles that speak to me at that moment.

Just like modifying the postures themselves so they best suit you, I encourage you to find your own tempo, pace, and schedule. Though I appreciate an eight-weeks-to or twenty-eight-days-to format for books and programs designed to motivate us, I see our progression of *awaken, transform*, and *unite* as ongoing and alive, as the architecture of every yoga practice, every relationship, every day, and every season of our constantly changing lives. I believe we have the opportunity to begin again and again, with every breath and in myriad situations. But you have to really do it. You have to climb out of the stands and onto the field.

We're going to find our way into a classic savasana pose and take some time to appreciate the inherent S.T.O.P. to S.T.A.R.T that lives within it.

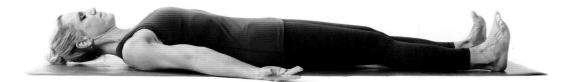

**Lie down on your back, arms along your sides but not glued to your ribs, legs a little bit wider than hip distance apart. Allow your feet to naturally fall open a bit. If your lower back is tender, you might prefer to bend your knees and put your feet on the ground. Snuggle your shoulder blades to melt down your back instead of riding up into your ears. Feel the back of your head and the backs of your hands heavy into the ground. Let your fingers crinkle toward your palms with relaxation. Appreciate the support of the earth beneath you, how it literally has your back, reinforcing safe surrender. Imagine your muscles turning into liquid and that liquid seeping into the floorboards beneath you, your bones sinking into the ground as if elementally returning to the earth. Yield to these bodily sensations and allow the blizzard of thoughts and stories in your snow globe head to succumb to the calm resolve. Reach full S.T.O.P.—body and mind.**

Stay here for five minutes using your timer or **@OM**.

## ON YOUR OM

We can S.T.O.P. to S.T.A.R.T. anywhere at any time—in your office when you're ready to strangle your boss, in your parked car after dropping off screaming kids, when you've tried in vain to reach an actual human being instead of an automated phone menu, or before starting a new project or task.

Begin by taking little S.T.O.P. to S.T.A.R.T. savasanas throughout the day. You don't have to take the actual pose like you did **On Your Mat** (though you're welcome to), but you will find your way toward the palpable calm you felt while in the posture. Sit without returning a text or e-mail, pause without planning, stand and close your eyes without seeing your shopping list . . . just for thirty seconds. Try to fit three in per day. Set your timer or use **@OM.** When you feel you are arriving at thirty seconds, try a full minute, then maybe even two. Notice how it stops the confusion and provides you with a new platform from which to start again. As Anne Lamott says, "Almost everything will work again if you unplug it for a few minutes, including you."

# 2

# Present vs. Tense

*There is never anything but the*

*present, and if one cannot live*

*there, one cannot live anywhere.*

—ALAN WATTS

**In this chapter you *awaken* to the fact that landing in the present moment is the recipe for stepping out of your own way and into the fullness of your life.**

Ask anyone "How are you?," and you're likely to get "busy" or " tired" as a response. In fact, we're so hopped up on hectic we've started to allow it to define not just how, but *who* we are. Our bodies and minds are held hostage by chronic stress. Stress is conflict between desire/expectation and current reality. When we S.T.O.P. to S.T.A.R.T. we begin to become present to what *is* instead of exhausting ourselves by ruminating on a past we cannot change or obsessively rehearsing for a future that isn't here yet. Breathing allows us to land in the present moment, get out of our own way, and build upon S.T.O.P. to S.T.A.R.T.

Let's take a look at how stress paralyzes us. Here's an example (you can find audio guidance for this exercise **@OM** too):

Imagine standing and squeezing your toes as tightly as you can. Keep squeezing them as you tense up the rest of your feet as much as possible without stopping. Let this rigidity travel up to your ankles and into your lower legs (keep squeezing your toes and feet!). Tense up your upper legs, your hips, your belly, your butt, and your back muscles. (How are those toes and feet doing?) Now curl up your fingers and hands into angry fists, tighten your forearms and upper arms too. Shrug your shoulders into your ears. Don't let any of the stiffness you've created dissipate. Squish up your neck and throat as well as your face. Let yourself become a gigantic stress ball and don't let one bit of it go! Without releasing any squeezing, try to lean forward and touch your toes . . . no, no don't loosen any of it . . .

It's impossible, right?

The intention is there, but the tension makes you a prisoner in your own body.

Now place your hands on your chest and feel your breath rise and fall. Envision that you have gills (I know, just stay with me) and that those gills are filling up and allowing you to breathe more and more deeply, bringing richer, smoother breaths into your body with each inhale and exhale. S.T.O.P. to S.T.A.R.T.—become present to where you are and what you're feeling right now, not what you think you should feel, or will feel, or have felt before. Sense the spaciousness of your inhales and the rooted, grounded calm of your exhales. Notice the shift in your body and how relaxation and ease (which remind you a lot of savasana) are replacing the stress and tension you just indulged. Powerful conscious breathing is the foundation of yoga and meditation practice. You can feel debilitating drama start to shift to the background and spacious possibility rise in your consciousness.

Remain here and experience the calm simplicity of your breathing for one minute. After a full minute, gently consider folding at the hips and reaching for your toes. Take note of how you've managed to get out of your own way. You may not actually get all that close to touching your toes, but this time you can definitely move toward your intention to do so.

Our breath is something we often take for granted. We breathe all the time unconsciously or else we wouldn't be alive. But for most of us this unconscious breathing is tense, erratic, and shallow. Certainly you bumped up against this in the exercise above. In yoga we refer to breath work as *pranayama*. Pranayama literally translates as "to extend vital life force," but don't let the lofty-sounding definition scare you off. Breathing is a tool accessible to us all that allows us to land in our body and to quiet our mind.

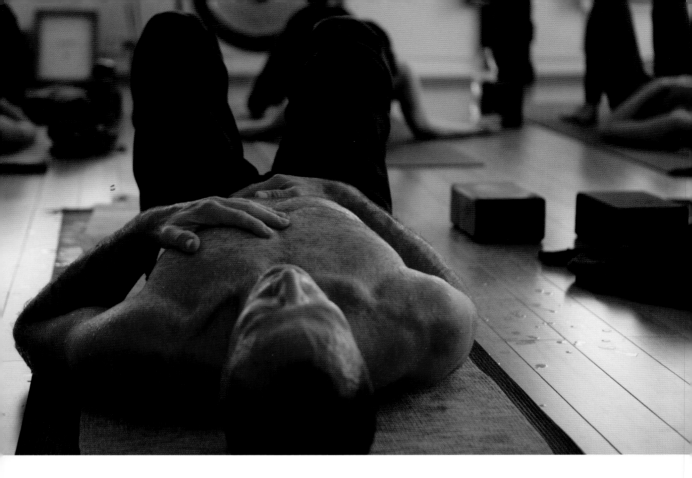

## ON YOUR MAT

Let's *awaken* to the fundamentals of our breathing. Even if yours is a steady diet of nadi shodhana (alternate nostril breathing) and kapalabahti (breath of fire), meet me here at the breath work ABCs:

**Awareness**

**Benevolence**

**Calm**

Lie on your back with your feet flat on the floor a little bit wider than hip distance apart. Let your knees knock in on one another so your lower back feels comfortable. Place your hands on your belly and notice your breath. Become **Aware**. That's all—just pay attention. Does your breath feel shallow? Choppy? Rushed? Do you favor your inhale or your exhale? As you take note, can you do so with **Benevolence** (kindness and grace) and allow yourself to relax into **Calm**? Can you feel your abdomen rise as you inhale and fall as you exhale? Are you able to let this rise and fall, slow down, deepen, and widen? Take a few moments here just to observe.

Now that you've discovered your ABCs lying on your back, you're going to add them to a bit of movement using a simple flow called Cat/Cow. Come onto your hands and knees. If your knees are unhappy here, pad them with a blanket or towel and/or feel free to keep your toes tucked under for more support.

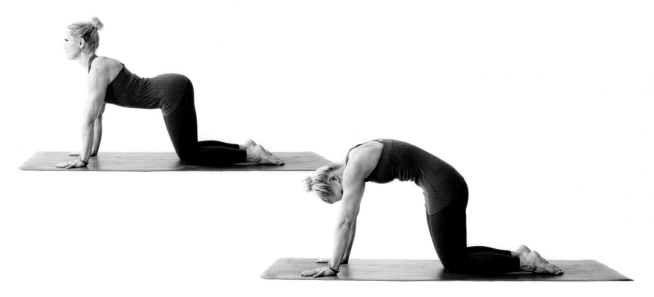

As you inhale, arch your back, pulling your chest through the gateway of your arms and lengthening your spine.

As you exhale, round and dome your back, drawing your belly toward your spine. Try it on for size, and then begin to find a rhythm—inhaling and exhaling, arching and contracting. Pay special attention to your breath and to how it facilitates **Awareness, Benevolence,** and **Calm** even amid this more dynamic movement. Allow the sensations of the postures to deepen your experience of the **ABCs.** As I'm sure you'll notice, Cat/Cow happens to be a delicious release for your tin-man spine and slumped-in-my-seat shoulders too. Appreciate how simple breathing and movement replenish and refresh from the inside out. **Awareness, Benevolence, Calm**—body, mind, spirit.

In addition to your daily practice of thirty-second S.T.O.P. S.T.A.R.T savasana pauses throughout the day, you'll add these ABCs when you first wake up in the morning and before you go to bed. It's super straightforward: S.T.O.P. to S.T.A.R.T., and then lie down and breathe into your ABCs for five minutes just like we did together above (you can even throw in a few Cat/Cows before if you'd like).

And yes, you have the time to do it. Wake up five minutes earlier and spend five fewer minutes perusing Amazon.com or the same headlines. This is the perfect thing to do while your coffee is brewing or your teakettle is heating up in the morning. Just decide you're going to stay clear of your computer or mobile screens (except for using @OM) until you're done with your five minutes. At night make this a non-negotiable part of your bedtime ritual. Lie down, on the floor or even on your bed, S.T.O.P., S.T.A.R.T., and breathe into Awareness, Benevolence, and Calm. It's that simple . . . but you have to really do it. Twice. Every day.

## ON YOUR OM

Earlier I encouraged you to modify your postures and find your own pace on your mat. The same is true of **On Your OM**. Each one of us will have our own unique self-actualization understanding as we make our way through our **Close to OM** journey together. It's taken me years to truly comprehend how to translate Present vs. Tense and ABCs from my mat to my life. . . . and to be honest I'm still working on it. These juicy foundational elements never get boring. They provide ongoing insight when the tension of the first exercise in this chapter infiltrates everyday trials and tribulations: the grocery line you're standing in isn't moving fast enough—your kid or mate still isn't listening when you ask them to make the bed—you take a business hiccup personally.

But then you *awaken*.

Out in the world it may not be instant, but from your work on your mat you remember to S.T.O.P., recognize your agitation, and become aware that you're tangled up in stress. This might be as far as you get for a while, and that's fabulous progress. If you're impatient, anxious that you should be able to S.T.A.R.T. right away, or tightly wound around how it's supposed to go from here, you'll only jam yourself deeper into your initial tension. When you find yourself at the eye of an emotional storm, observe what's happening. Just notice. Like you did on your mat.

Next, step into your office, the other room, or somewhere conducive to placing your hands on your chest, as we did at the beginning of the chapter to witness the rise and fall of your breath. Is it choppy? Shallow? Rushed? Are you able to convince it to slow and deepen? Envision yourself lying in the ease of savasana (in fact, lie down on the ground and actually do it if it's helpful and doable where you are). Can you be here with your breath instead of seduced by dizzying empirical drama? Getting to this point is its own breakthrough and incredible evidence that your **On Your Mat** discovery is spilling into your life.

Integrating ABCs in real-time is rich terrain. Accessing Awareness, Benevolence, and Calm can feel a bit elusive simply lying on our back for five minutes every day, don't you think? Realizing these ABCs amid the chaos of life's ups and downs is to be truly Present vs. Tense. Your increasing sense of Awareness opens you up to a pocket of space like we experienced together in the second part of our tension exercise. From this space Benevolence can blossom, allowing you to trade in a mind-set that is compulsive for one that is compassionate—interested instead of impulsive. You begin to understand that freaking out is not going to get the line to move any faster, skyrocketing your adrenaline will not get the bed made, and taking things personally when they aren't is bad business all around. Instead of catastrophizing imaginary scenarios, you become clear about what's actually happening, and can drop into a quieter sense of Calm.

Over time these steps may become more seamless and immediate for you. There are moments when the process is concurrent for me, and others when I'm grateful for the bit-by-bit progression deconstructed above. Both methods are tools in my real-life toolbox only because I continue to practice them every day on my mat. Just like you . . . right?

# 3

# To Begin, *Begin*

*In the beginner's mind there*

*are many possibilities, but in*

*the expert's there are few.*

—ZEN MASTER SHUNRYO SUZUKI

**In this chapter you *awaken* to the fact that in order to live into your full potential and the life you want, you must be willing to become a beginner again.**

"My goal is to have a goal." One of my students told me the other day. "My job sucks, I'm tired all the time. I can't motivate myself to date anyone. I'm sick of being sick of myself. I need to do something and I don't know where to start."

Can you relate? I sure can.

The fact that you've picked up this book gives me a sneaking suspicion that perhaps, in your own way, your goal is to have a goal too. But how can we possibly have a goal or a vision if we can't see beyond our own fog? We need a guiding light to get us through the haze. So many good intentions wither before they can ever bear fruit. Diets disappear into midmorning chocolate-covered almonds on the very first day. Projects are left abandoned, like forgotten unmatched socks. We keep clocking in at the same job, wallowing in the same disappointment, and wondering why nothing ever changes even though we're desperate for a different result.

That period of my life when I first started yoga was a neurotic quest for more, more, more. *Nothing* was ever enough: no workout, no amount of success, no expression of love, nothing. I managed to turn everything into a letdown. I was restless, impatient, and had decided that I was horribly lonely. That was my story and I was sticking to it.

What story are you sticking to?

Though I spent hours at Crunch Gym spinning and stepping and God knows what else, I had no interest in yoga until I stumbled into class one evening convinced it wasn't going to burn enough calories to be worthwhile. I mostly remember the nausea. I couldn't seem to manage the simplest instruction, was completely irritated by the pace of the class and by the teacher who kept reminding me not to fidget. Between waves of nausea, though, I could feel something important calling, something radically contrary to my insatiable need for more.

There's something confrontational about that first down dog. Yes, we are inverting our heart and hips above our head, and strengthening and stretching muscles we didn't realize we even had. But that's not all. We can feel that we've stepped into something deeper than we realized, like walking out into the surf and suddenly finding an unexpected drop beneath our feet. Off-balance in this new terrain, we have to find courage, footing, and patience. Without courage, we will slither back to what is familiar and comfortable. Without patience we will find ourselves overwhelmed and giving up.

In this book, yoga's combination of physical, psychological, and philosophical discovery is our path to the other side of stuck. Think of it as our GPS to help us identify exactly where it is that we're inhibited so we can move through and then beyond it to a space of possibility, inspiration, originality, resourcefulness, and vision.

Awakening is the first step. We have to *awaken* to what's really going on. In other words we have to get out from underneath that story we've been sticking to. Chances are that's going to challenge and even annoy you at times, as it did me. Which is where the courage and patience I mentioned comes in. But, rest assured, ultimately we're going to have fun making our way **Close to OM** and using yoga to create a life we love.

There's a saying that we begin again every time we step onto our mat. So whether you are brand-new and literally stepping onto your mat for the first time, or years into your yoga practice, we are all essentially beginners together. The beauty of being a beginner is the "beginner's mind." The mind of a beginner is one that is open and ready to learn. It's not bogged down with what it thinks it already knows. There is newness to everything.

Our yoga GPS "technology" is thousands of years old. And within that technology is evidence that seeking a wide-open beginner's mind in the face of our stories and excuses is nothing new to us humans. The Bhagavad Gita is a sacred Hindu scripture and an important historical yogic text written sometime between the fifth and second century BCE. Part of the larger Mahabharata, it is the conversation between Krishna and Arjuna before the start of the Kurukshetra war. From a yogic point of view, it addresses the tension between our easily distracted senses and our intuition, as well as how we view our place in the world as an individual versus a being unified with all. It is an exploration of how to balance Self (*Atman*) and the Supreme Being (*Bhagavan*). Mahatma Gandhi says of the Gita, "It is an allegory in which the battlefield is the soul and Arjuna, man's higher impulses, struggling against evil."

In our own way, as we climb onto our mat for the first time, we are like Arjuna, grappling with our own unfortunate tendencies (hopefully they are more bothersome than they are "evil") and suddenly being asked to focus in ways we have never done. We find that there are myriad emotions involved in trying to create stillness amid physical challenge, and to staving off the distractions of our impulsive minds. It doesn't help that our ego is tap dancing wildly nearby, hopped up on self-absorption, thumb to its nose as we do our best to follow instructions without feeling too foolish or clumsy. Not to mention that we've become addicted to swinging from instant messaging to instant checkout to Instagram to insta-alarmist sound bites and back again like monkeys swinging from branch to branch. In this jungle of immediate and often vapid "communication," it is easy to lose sight of anything higher, larger, or universal.

So there it all is, up in our face in our downward facing dog.

Ultimately, yoga is an experience, not a discussion. It's not artificial or self-involved; instead it is honest in ways we may not like to hear. It is, as we sense in that first dog, larger than the poses, and it tells us who we really are, like it or not. It is an opportunity for us to realize that it's more fulfilling to do the work than it is to avoid it. It asks us to dig ourselves out from under all our chaos and agitation and create a real blossom, not a showy synthetic one. It is the quintessential moment, breath by breath, for us to witness that how we do one thing is how we do everything. The way we operate on our mat is the same as we do off of it.

So, as if Krishna were whispering in *our* ear, let's muster the courage to move forward together and to find the kind of patience within us that will allow our potential to expand more than we could have imagined.

In other words, let's begin.

## ON YOUR MAT

Prepare to climb into downward facing dog (adho mukha svanasana), but before you do, prepare to begin again. Even if you're an old pro convinced you've got this dog nailed and can do it blindfolded with your hands tied behind your back. Even if you've done a bazillion of them, imagine this is your first down dog ever, and you are feeling it in such a way as to describe every nuance to someone who won't get the chance to do one of their own. You're going to try to stay here for five minutes, which sounds like nothing until it's your turn to do it. You'll set your timer or use @OM. Curl your toes under, lift your hips up and back, and turn your body into an inverted V shape.

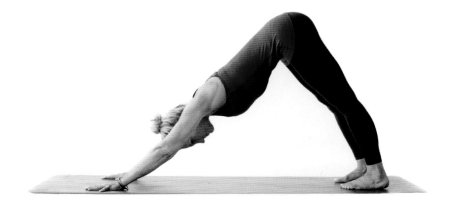

**In downward facing dog, spread your hands wide, shoulder distance apart on your mat, careful to press down into the index finger and thumb and not let them crinkle up with tension or neglect. Think of it as reaching all of your fingers into**

deep rich soil. Imagine a circle around the circumference of your palm and try to maintain the imprint of that entire circle. Let your forearms draw toward one another and lift away from the ground, creating strong, straight arms. Allow your head to hang fully relaxed between your arms, lining up your ears with your biceps. Encourage your shoulder blades away from your neck and away from each other, as if cascading off the sides of your torso and taking your stresses along with them. Notice how determined they are to climb up into your ears. Lift your sit bones to the sky and descend your heels to the ground; enjoy a release through the backs of your legs and an elongation along the entire length of your spine. Part forward fold, part gentle inversion (hips inverted over heart), even the physical shape of down dog suggests a contemplative inward turn and a shift in perspective.

I know that you won't need to—not you, you've totally got this—but if someone needed to come out of this early they absolutely could . . . You might try closing your eyes to help turn the arrows of attention away from any distractions outside too.

To be clear, this is not an indulgent foot-pedaling, bouncy, leg-lifting puppy dog—it's four on the floor, nothing more. Be willing to be still. Pay close attention to where your body meets the ground as well as how it lifts and extends away from the pull of gravity. Are resistance or impatience bubbling up and limiting your perception of newness? Can you set them aside and return to the many possibilities of your beginner's mind, as our Zen Master Suzuki quote at the top of the chapter suggests? Or are you the stoic "expert" he mentions whose possibilities are "few"?

While you're in down dog beginning again, are you breathing? Are your wrists sore? Is there tightness anywhere? Is it stretch or strength that you notice most? Where? Can you make one brand-new discovery about your down dog that you've never noticed before? It might be a physical sensation or even an emotional response. Just like you're practicing sprinkling little savasanas throughout your day, ideally you add an element of peaceful savasana surrender to every pose. Can you manage that here, even in the midst of this dynamic dog?

Down dog is that pause in vinyasa yoga where you take inventory of how and what you are feeling in that particular moment. Where you check in with your breath and reestablish your focus. It is the end of one vinyasa and the beginning of another. The awareness we cultivate in down dog informs the rest of our practice, our Self, and ultimately our life. Pausing to pay attention to subtleties creates conscious space for something new. Our bodies become unstuck along with our minds and we can access our beginner's mind again and again.

## ON YOUR OM

What we do on our mat is merely a reflection of how we function off our mat. Maybe you sensed a bit of my punishing "nothing's ever enough" as you held your down dog. Or perhaps your thing is to give up before even trying. We may feel immovably weak or fearful, inadequate, or just set like cement in what we think we know. None of this means that we're disappointing or lazy or bad; my point is this stuff doesn't live in a vacuum. How we do our yoga is how we do our life. What happens in a yoga pose provides incredible insight into our behaviors, relationships, and choices even after we roll up our mats.

As you make your way through this book, whether the information is an introduction or more of a review, I encourage you to read it with your beginner's mind. If you've been at this yoga thing for a while, take a step back from the strict drishti (established gazing points), alignment obsessions, and physical accomplishments you may have acquired along the way and find a moment to reflect on your first yoga experience. Pause, and remember how wonderfully naïve you were not knowing what would happen and how.

There is inspiring freedom when we pause and begin again. We become present to things that may have been eclipsed by our shuffle—how refreshing it is to listen and actually hear, how insightful it is to linger in the scope of a question without needing to provide the answer, how extraordinary it is to experience the subtle textures of new light. To *awaken* is to see that the beginning is invariably today, and the present moment is the doorway to the infinite.

View your daily routines through this beginner's mind aperture and become fascinated by what might have become mundane. Like your little savasanas throughout the day, I'm going to ask you to pay close attention. Start as you wake up to a new day. Note the things you do each morning that you usually don't pay any attention to. Stop and actually appreciate the smell and taste of your coffee or tea. Take in the sounds, the temperature, the color of the sky, your cat begging for treats, husband snoring in the other room—allow these perceptions to turn repetition into ritual and disinterest into discovery.

What if I were to tell you that truly "advanced" yoga is not about what elaborate tricks you can pull out of your sleeve or how flexible your body is—it's the awareness and integrity with which you do the simplest of things. Your beginner's mind is your introduction to radical transformation. And the crazy part is, radical transformation comes from subtle shifts.

# 4

# Inquire Within

*A man who as a physical being is always turned toward the outside, thinking that his happiness lies outside him, finally turns inward and discovers that the source is within him.*

—SØREN KIERKEGAARD

**In this chapter, you *awaken* to how S.T.O.P. to S.T.A.R.T., your ABCs of breathing, and your beginner's mind lead you to pratyahara—an inward instead of distractedly outward turn—for answers.**

After my first down dog, no confetti dropped from the sky. No one handed me a huge oversize check or diploma and congratulated me, but things were shifting and I was adjusting in ways that were subtle but significant. There may not have been a tickertape parade after that initial dog, but there *was* a lightning bolt of sorts. I realized that the vulnerability I was feeling in my life was like the vulnerability I felt in that nauseating dog. It occurred to me that maybe the tools my time spent on my mat was giving me might be useful to deconstruct my off-mat challenges too. And that gave me the guts to sign up for a teacher training. I devoured the syllabus and read the Bhagavad Gita,

Patanjali's *Yoga Sutras*, Beryl Bender Birch's *Power Yoga*, *The Heart of Yoga*, *Hatha Yoga Pradipika*, *The Tree of Yoga*, *Light on Yoga*, anything I could get my hands on.

It turned out that the asana (poses) I'd been learning so much from were just the tip of the iceberg. There were *eight* limbs to the tree of yoga, and asana was only one of them. The others were: yama (universal morality), niyama (personal observances), pranayama (breath work), pratyahara (withdrawal of the senses), dharana (concentration), dhyana (meditation), and samadhi (total immersion into pure unfiltered consciousness).

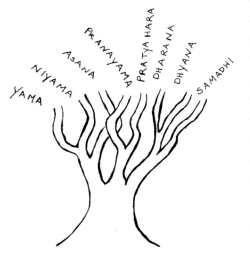

My teacher training was at a little local studio located in a strip mall between tanning and hair extension salons. Like political propaganda, banners and flags with the little local studio owners' self-assigned yoga name and signature long-haired silhouette were everywhere. "He's the best" quotes from random celebrities were situated at eye-level so as not to be missed, and clothing emblazoned with his brand was his uniform even away from the studio. He was quite sought after by the ladies, who outnumbered the men fifteen to one in our teacher training class. I am forever grateful for the inestimable lessons I learned during my tenure in his kingdom. Some of which were not part of the intended curriculum.

It turns out every one of us, regardless of our "practice random acts of kindness" bumper stickers, has an ego to wrestle with, and my local teacher/trainer was no exception. Like a pair of sunglasses you can't find that are perched right on top of your head, he seemed to have a little trouble locating the yogic ideology he was advocating when he needed it for himself. Distracted by his adoring audience, technical issues with the video camera he'd set up to capture his lecture, and whether to pull his hair into a ponytail or not, he began our lesson:

"Pratyahara is a withdrawal of the senses," he told us, glancing at the video monitors. "When the mind is guided by wandering senses, then it carries away one's understanding, as does the wind a ship on the water." He quoted from the Bhagavad Gita while indicating an adjusted camera angle to the work-study student behind the lens. "This fifth limb in Patanjali's *Yoga Sutras* asks us to draw our awareness away from outside stimuli or the external world and turn quietly inward."

It was at that moment I realized he was a mirror of my own turbulent tendencies. Tossed about by superficial agitation, none of us can dive deep enough to get beneath our whirlpools of thought and commotion. His was the perfect presentation for me to grasp that pratyahara is a state of consciousness, not just an intellectual concept. It *awakens* us to the gnosis of our true self instead of the clamor of stories we tell ourselves, distractions we indulge, or personas we perpetuate. Pratyahara allows us to pay attention to a more intuitive voice and prepare for concentration (dharana) and meditation (dhyana).

A super-helpful illustration of this for me is that pratyahara is absorbed through the subtle layers of the Self, our five sheaths, called koshas. From the ancient Hindu texts known as the Upanishads, they are:

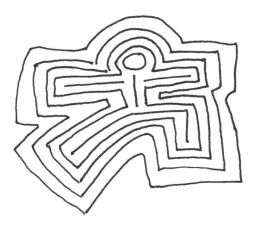

**annamaya kosha** (our outermost layer, skin and bones)

**pranamaya kosha** (energy channels)

**manomaya kosha** (*manas* means "mind"; the mental and emotional)

**vijnanamaya kosha** (wisdom, intellect as well as ego)

**anandamaya kosha** (*ananda* means "bliss"; it is the innermost, Soul, Atman, absolute, truth, Source)

Imagine them like the layers of an onion, or those little Russian dolls that fit inside one another and represent nature's five elements within us: earth, fire, water, air, and ether. Our outermost layer of skin and bones (annamaya kosha) is most tangible, which is what makes the poses a particularly immediate entry point for most of us. Pratyahara asks that we pare down the kerfuffle from our bodies (like we experienced in our tension exercise at the beginning of the book), as well as our minds, emotions, and ego so that we can land in the absolute truth of our soul body (anandamaya kosha).

When we feel frustrated or uninspired we often waste our energy searching for scape-goats and excuses. If we focus on everything and everyone else, we don't have to look at ourselves. On our mat that can show up as endlessly fixing . . . our shirt, our mat, our props, our pedicure (I've had someone get up off their mat and go to their purse to check their lipstick)—just to avoid the stretch or stillness of a pose. Off our mat our distractions and excuses ambush communication, connection, conversation, conviction, commitment, courage . . . and that's just one letter of the alphabet.

In fact, brahmancharya (control of the senses) is one of the yamas on our Eight-Limbed path, and in many ways an extension of pratyahara. In the texts we studied in my teacher trainings, brahmancharya mostly had to do with decorum and being considerate. The larger thesis is one of respect and not wasting our divine energy on that which is irresponsible. Think of it as keeping oil in your lamp so as not to burn out. There are, however, more extreme examples of the concept of brahmancharya as self-imposed celibacy for the sake of spiritual growth. The information out there about sex and yoga can be pretty misleading. Tantra, which we hear so much about, for example, is more of a spiritual science than it is a sex cult or an ancient set of instructions as to how to perform bendy orgies. Tantra is a style of practice that uses meditation, mantra, and prana (life force energy) to attain spiritual and even mystical liberation. It uses the physical body as a tool to reach the more subtle layers of the Self. Yes, sometimes in relation to sex, but not nearly as often or in the same ways as *Cosmo* magazine would have you believe.

Pratyahara is a vital component of yoga philosophy. It's an inward, not outward, turn— the practice of *not* being distracted. Listening to our breath instead of the sound of an incoming text message. Clearing our minds of the chitta vritti (whirlpools of thought) that keep us looking frantically outside for answers that lie within. With pratyahara we build on our beginner's mind and breath work. It's a way to consistently concentrate our energy on what matters and not be sabotaged by what doesn't. We cannot *awaken* to personal progress if we aren't committed to our inward turn.

## ON YOUR MAT

Tadasana (mountain pose) is the bedrock of asana. Most every pose has tadasana within it, and in vinyasa-style sequencing, tadasana offers a moment of pause and reflection. I often cue to my class "return to your mountain" as we come into tadasana. A mountain sits regardless of season, weather, hikers digging their heels in, or skiers scraping its surface. Stepping into our own inner mountain allows us a place to S.T.O.P. and S.T.A.R.T. and shift from preoccupation to pratyahara throughout the ebb and flow of our practice and our lives.

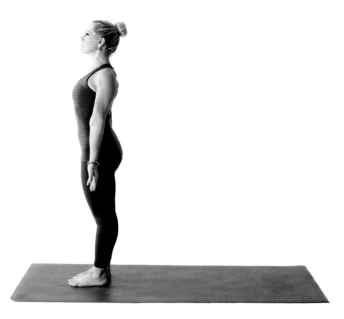

**Standing with your feet hip distance apart (or if you prefer, big toes touching and heels a few inches apart), place your hands on your chest as we did after our tension exercise, and witness the rise and fall of your breath. Weave in the Awareness, Benevolence, and Calm of the ABCs you've been practicing as you breathe. After about thirty seconds here, either bring your hands into a prayer in front of your chest or let your arms release along the sides of your body. If you're bringing your arms alongside you, some people will tell you to face your palms toward your body, others will ask you to spin your palms forward to invite external rotation and less internal habitual slump to your shoulders. I'm going to have you open your palms forward to encourage a lift to your chest and wide collarbones as you see in this photo. If your hands are in a prayer imagine elevating your sternum (chest bone) into your prayer.**

Begin by observing your connection to the earth. Note whether you're favoring one side over the other—right and left, or one aspect of your foot—front/back/inside/outside.

Create an expansive base and sense the length of all your toes, solid big toe and pinky toe knuckles and the points on both your inner and outer heels as they connect to the floor. Find samasthiti, which means "even standing" and is actually another name for tadasana. Allow your inhales to lift the crown of your head to the sky and your exhales to surrender your foundation deeper into the ground. As you stand here, centered and grounded in what's almost an upright savasana, the outside world buzzes and swirls around you. People come and go, clouds pass, and the sun creates shadows and light. Yet your mountain remains unwavering in its stillness. The inward turn of pratyahara *awakens* you to a panoramic view that is deeply internal and vastly universal all at once.

Like you did with down dog earlier, you are going to stand in tadasana for five minutes. What could be easier, right? I mean who can't just stand there for five minutes? In case you're convinced you're too advanced for this tadasana exercise, allow me to reintroduce you to your beginner's mind. If I may be so bold, this mountain is an ascent especially designed for those of us who think we don't need it. I only know because that was my attitude when I first bumped up against this new altitude too.

Try to use a way of keeping time that doesn't lend itself to restless fuss and constant checking—something you don't need to look at until it gently chimes you to climb out of your mountain—something that facilitates instead of inhibits pratyahara exploration. Of course using @OM is perfect for this—there I'll guide you through *and* keep the time for you all at once.

You're going to reassume the stance described above. If you can manage closing your eyes here without falling over, that would be fabulous; gazing softly toward the ground in front of you works just fine as well. You'll invite your ABCs to your mountain again and again. And you'll note seismic waves of potential interruption attempting to call your bluff as you decide to stay.

Initially it's as if you've wandered onto your mountain in the dark and it takes a moment to adjust to the obscurity. Then, if you allow them to, your breath and the sensations you're experiencing shine light upon your landscape. First the dawn is dim, but as you remain, the sky opens up and you can begin to make out the details of a nuanced path toward peace.

Once you've stepped off the elevation of your five-minute mountain, I'm going to give you a grounding exercise that builds upon your ABCs and assists pratyahara. We're going to move from incline to supine.

After you read through this description of what we're up to next, you'll set your timer or use @OM to immerse yourself in it for three undisturbed minutes.

You'll lie on your back, knees bent, feet hip distance apart and flat on the floor, and begin to breathe just through your nose. Place your hands on your belly and feel it rise on the inhale and fall on the exhale. Take note. If your inhales are longer than your exhales, see if you can gently shift toward making the two sides even. If you are able to arrive at even breathing (sama vritti), begin to make your exhales a bit longer than your inhales—eventually moving toward a 2 to 1 ratio. Don't be overly ambitious. Even just a slightly longer exhale is perfect. Feel the relaxation of the exhales and how they make your body feel heavy into the ground—less agitated and restless. Try silently telling yourself "let" as you inhale, and "go" as you exhale, and allow this to persuade you to surrender further.

Our nervous system is the communication center of our bodies. It's where our inside world interacts with and interprets the outside world. Your exhales are inspiring what's called the relaxation response in your nervous system. It's the flip side of the stress response, or what you might know as "fight or flight." We need the stress response for our survival. It's a shot of adrenaline that gets us out of the way of danger (think oncoming bus). It shuts down systems like our digestion and immune system that we would need later, raises our blood pressure, and funnels all our energy and resources toward high alert: *"Get me out of here now!"* It's like the gas pedal for our nervous system.

Problems occur when we keep our foot on the gas and our engines idle in this high alert. Those systems we now need are compromised and the ill effects on our health are what we know as chronic stress, or distress. High blood pressure, digestion problems, weight gain, insomnia, anxiety, and many other issues can result from keeping our foot on the gas when it is no longer needed. Chronic stress has won itself the title of "number one killer" in many medical dialogues. Our distracted minds are fuel for chronic stress, and pratyahara helps us take our foot off the gas and move it to the brake.

I'd like you to try to breathe with these extended exhales as part of the five-minute ABCs you're doing every morning and evening like a little visceral reminder of your peaceful mountain. Feel them as a furthering tool to add pratyahara to Awareness, Benevolence, and Calm, and to touch base with your relaxation response. Drop out of your stressed-out, distracted state and onto your path toward holistic understanding.

Continue to take your little savasanas throughout the day too. Oh, and how's it going with the "pay close attention" we talked about? Are you noticing the ingredients of your life in ways that continue to shift repetition into ritual and disinterest into discovery? Have you been taking time to truly taste—to not just hear but to listen—to see what's hiding under your haste? Are you beginning to *awaken* to the mountain of insight that comes from the groundwork you're doing? Pausing, paying attention, and looking inward with Awareness, Benevolence, and Calm cultivate soil in which seeds of change can grow.

## ON YOUR OM

As a means to move your mountain off your mat, I'm going to ask you to do something fundamental and oddly profound. Choose an afternoon to leave your phone at home. Not an afternoon when you're anticipating an important call from your boss or when your kid is sick and might need to reach you. Pick an afternoon that looks free and clear so that you can become free and clear. Oh, and while you're at it, log off of your computer and take that iPad out of your bag too. What I'm asking for is a minimum of three hours of no technology. (Once upon a time nobody had cell phones and yet they left their houses and went about their lives . . . hard to believe, I know.) There are many ways in which technology enhances our lives, but allowing us to turn quietly inward is not one of them. I like the analogy that technology is like fire. We can cook, warm ourselves, and even create light with fire. But if we misuse it we may end up burning ourselves.

Allow me to go out on a limb here and suggest that perhaps I'm not the only one who occasionally burns herself with her technology. You know how it is. The sound of our in-box becomes so provocative that we can't possibly keep both hands on the wheel, or finish reading the chapter, or stay tuned-in to the conversation we're having. Like an obedient robot we reach for our iPhone and enter our passcode without missing a beat. And that reminds us that we haven't checked to see if anyone liked or commented on the Facebook post we put up. Which in turn has us wondering how many followers we're up to on Twitter. And crap, we never picked a filter for that picture of the glass of water we just had, and down the rabbit hole we go . . . Right?

Consider your phoneless afternoon a counterpose to this technology-driven madness. Go for a walk. Have actual face time with a friend as opposed to FaceTime. Enjoy a meal without distraction, head to the museum or to the park. Paint, draw, dance, sing, cook, fold laundry, garden, read an actual book with real pages, get a massage, sit and look at the ocean, a sunset, your children, the grass growing. . . just don't log on to anything.

If you're like me, it's a bit shocking just how embedded the desire is to reach for the phone or sit in front of the computer. There are days when the Yoga Police might revoke my license if they saw how impulsively attached I'd been. Our awakening is an ongoing process and our samskara (habits) can be very sly and determined. Just as we begin again every time we step onto our mat, we begin over and over again as we start to become familiar with how our mind works.

How we do our yoga is how we do our life.

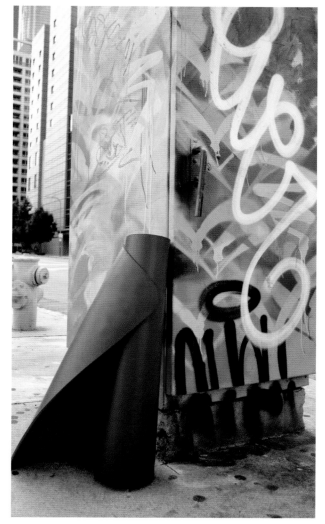

When I feel myself buried in a technological quagmire, I give myself the same assignment I have given to you. Ideally I extend the afternoon to last over a day or even several days. I find that easiest to do when I am on a retreat. And I observe the same decompression in the students who come with me. It usually takes us about twenty-four hours of withdrawal until we land offline and in paradise. With Wi-Fi pretty much everywhere, this has become something increasingly difficult for me to enforce, but as you'll experience during your afternoon, it is incredibly necessary. In order to find our way inward, we have to turn down the outside noise—and we start by turning it all the way off.

# 5

# Clearing the Way

*Clarity is the most important thing. I compare clarity to pruning in gardening. If you're not clear, nothing is going to happen.*

**—DIANE VON FURSTENBERG**

**In this chapter you *awaken* to the need to create an internal and external environment conducive to positive change.**

Our environment is a reflection of our mind. If we are careless and unfocused mentally, that's what we're creating and perpetuating. The yogic tenet saucha (cleanliness/purity) can help us establish a clean, clear, conducive canvas for our beginner's mind and an inward turn to move us beyond being stuck in our chaos and funk. And the makings of chaos and funk are everywhere—not just in your kid's closet, husband's man cave, or creepy overflowing recycling bin.

Never have I had such a response to a newsletter I sent out to my student base like I did the time when I asked everyone to be conscious about hygiene and tidiness. Frantic e-mails poured in: "*I'm the one you were talking about, right?*" People cornered me before and after class, whispering like they were in a confessional: *I was doing a liver cleanse and I thought no one would notice.* New mats and outfits were purchased. Paranoia perfumed the landscape, along with freshly laundered yogitoes, towels, and breath mints, until I realized I needed to make something clear: the bouquet of yoga room offenses is rich and broad, but not one of us is exempt from contributing to the potpourri. That's right. *No one.* Our bodies are wonderful, complicated, and sometimes obstinate. Who hasn't had bad breath at one time or another? Whose armpits haven't smelled less than fresh? And sometimes we contribute to the bad odors out of forgetfulness. I call them the "should haves." As in "I should have washed that mat after last practice," or "I should have washed *me* after last practice or that greasy meal," or "I should have avoided the garlic at lunch" (or perhaps those beans).

Lest you think this chapter is merely going to devolve into the equivalent of six-year-olds telling fart jokes on the playground, I'm actually addressing one of the yogic "moral" codes. Saucha is part of the niyamas (observances) branch of the eight limbs on our yoga tree. Saucha is purity, cleanliness, and the inner disciplines and responsibilities required to achieve them. A great deal of the focus is on internal purification, diet, pranayama (breath work), and thought (ridding ourselves of resentments, prejudices, and anger). But even the seemingly superficial discussion of hygiene fits into this category. Our environment is a reflection of our mind. If we are careless and disordered mentally, that will reflect in our environment being dirty, untidy, and uncared for. When our environment is out of order and soiled, we have not created a surrounding that supports the clear, uncluttered focus that our yoga encourages us to find.

If you stumble in to your yoga class, stomach full, mat smelling of a thousand stinky feet, and a towel that you found marinating in the trunk of your car, still damp from last practice, saucha is not only impossible for you, it is made very difficult for those around you. When you create thoughtful space for yourself, you then extend that to others. Whether in the classroom or out in your life, how can you expect to make a clean break toward something fresh and new if you don't first take responsibility for cleaning up your side of the street? Like brushing your teeth before eating Oreos or smoking a cigarette after filling your lungs with fresh air on your morning hike, you can't keep creating roadblocks through your inattention and hope to move toward something better. The accountability of saucha clears the way to personal transformation.

# ON YOUR MAT

We're going to link together our down dog and mountain pose to create a little flow known as sun salutation A (surya namaskar A). Yes there are surya Bs and even Cs, but we are going to focus on As here. (Check out appendix 2 if you're curious about Bs and Cs.) Cobra (or for some of you, upward dog) and chaturanga (low pushup) will be joining us as part of the choreography. The movements of plank, to chaturanga, into upward dog (or cobra), and then down dog are referred to as a vinyasa. Yoga practices that incorporate these movements into their sequencing are known as vinyasa-style classes. But vinyasa also means "breath guiding the movement" and "placed in a deliberate and special way," which doesn't necessarily have anything to do with chaturanga/up dog/down dog . . . Are you still with me?

It could be argued that breath guides our movements as we make our way through our lives too. And certainly "placed in a deliberate and special way" sits nicely next to the "pay close attention" you are doing off your mat, right? Vinyasa is another little reminder that how we do our yoga is how we do our life. Every sun salutation A has a vinyasa within it.

First I'm going break down the poses for you below. Then you'll do the sequence two separate times under very different circumstances. You'll need to take some time in between attempts to create the contrasting situations I'll lay out for you, so some of you might even choose to do these on different days.

Begin by standing in tadasana (mountain pose) within the first foot or so of your mat. Pause, S.T.O.P to S.T.A.R.T, and find samasthiti (even standing) and sama vritti (even breathing). See if you can narrow your breathing down to through your nose instead of your mouth. I'm going to introduce you to ujjayi breathing. That's a catch at the back of your throat, which sounds a little bit like you're fogging a mirror with your mouth closed. It's not over-the-top Darth Vader huffing and puffing as if to prove mirror-domination— nor is it moaning and groaning like you're perpetually in the throes of passion. Just a soft, hollow whisper that you and perhaps someone right next to you (not down the hall) can hear. In fact, to me the ujjayi style of breathing is as much about experiencing texture as it is about creating sound. The feeling of air brushing against the back of your throat provides another instrument through which you can appreciate cadence and rhythm—

almost like internal music or a mantra. Again, there's no pressure to perform, just give it a shot. Stay here for a few minutes. Your arms can rest at your sides, or you can join them in a prayer in front of your heart.

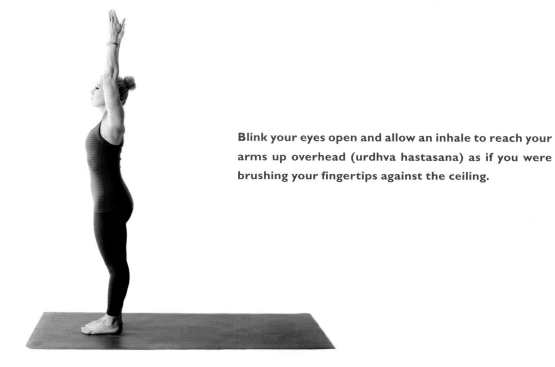

Blink your eyes open and allow an inhale to reach your arms up overhead (urdhva hastasana) as if you were brushing your fingertips against the ceiling.

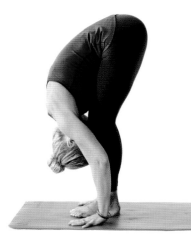

Exhale and fold at the hips, swan diving forward. Feel a gentle corseting action in your core supporting your lower back and hamstrings as you fold in chin toward the shins. Turn on the muscles in your legs by adding a bit of bend to your knees. Pay close attention so that you're not locking or forcing into your knees or creating sharp pain anywhere.

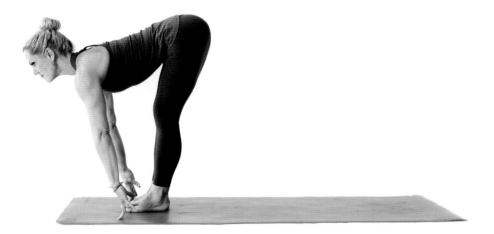

Inhale and look halfway up, extending your heart forward. Align fingertips next to your toes, or perhaps hands on the sides of the shins or a set of blocks for those of us on the tighter side. Exhale, and fold back in.

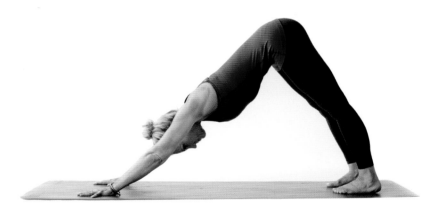

Just step one foot and then the other back to downward facing dog for our first round. Take six full cycles of breath here and nurture your sense of pratyahara (inward turn).

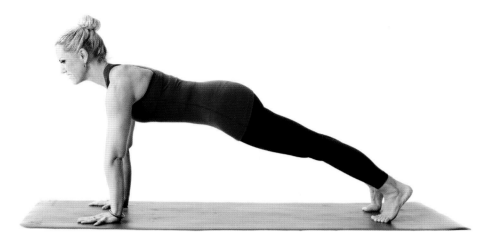

**Inhale into plank (upper pushup position).**

We're going to hang out here for a while, so you might prefer to put your knees down like a kickstand to buffer the physical intensity. A bit of fire is fine, but you never want physical ferocity to eclipse your ability to find deep, expansive breaths and little breezes of savasana. Your physical edge will show up differently every time you practice, so pay close attention (like you've been doing off your mat) to what makes sense for you right now. Don't confuse struggle with strength. I'd like you to stay here in your plank or modified plank for three to six full cycles of breath and then head back to your down dog for six full cycles of breath.

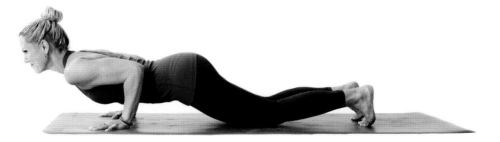

**Once again, inhale into plank, this time placing your knees down a little bit farther back in space than when we did with our Cat/Cow earlier.**

**With your gaze a bit forward and your core-corset intact, begin to bend your elbows toward a low pushup (chaturanga). Keep your elbows close enough to**

your body that they brush but don't crush your ribs—think aerodynamic vs. floppy-out-to-the-side wings. Try to keep your belly off the ground for three to six cycles of breath—then lower down onto your stomach (unless you happen to be pregnant).

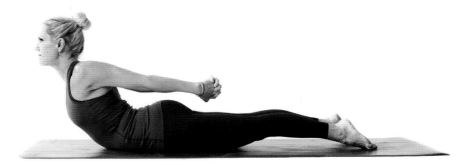

Face down, interlace your hands just above your butt, or hold a strap or towel to afford yourself more space. As if standing on your hip bones, begin to lengthen into a backbend (shalabhasana). Drag your interlaced knuckles toward the back edge of your mat and encourage your chest and rib cage to extend toward the front edge, as they gently lift up off of your mat. Press down into the tops of your feet and energize your legs so much that your kneecaps (but not your feet) lift off the ground. Resist the temptation to whiplash into the neck. Let this be less about tossing your chin forward and more about appreciating the feeling of the imprint of your shoulder blades into your spine. Smile your collarbones away from the ground as you counteract hours of slumping behind the wheel and collapsing at your desk. Think elongating as opposed to hoisting high when it comes to your backbend. Your tailbone lengthens toward your feet, creating more and more distance between your bottom ribs and pelvis, as if administering a thoughtful dose of therapeutic traction. Stay here for three to six full cycles of breath and then release and make a pillow with your hands, resting your head to one side.

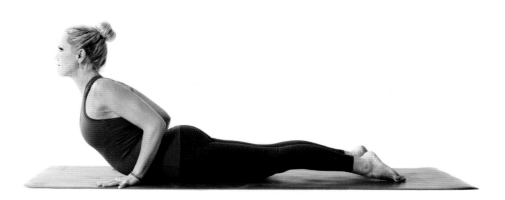

**Remain on your belly and position your hands next to your floating ribs like you did in your chaturanga (low pushup). Keep your aerodynamic wings (elbows stay close toward your body) as you pull your chest through the gateway of your arms for cobra (bhujangasana).**

The energy of your arms feels almost as if you were attempting to drag yourself off the front of your mat. Sense an imaginary interlace behind your back continuing to inform your long, sleek, spinal extension—no crunching, no flinging, just finessing and elongating.

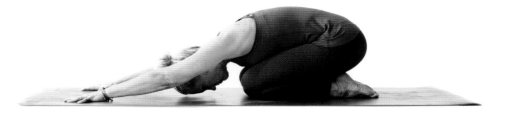

**From your cobra, shift your hips back to sit on your heels for child's pose (balasana).**

Arms can continue to reach out in front of you as they were in your down dog or you can run them alongside your body as if reaching for your heels. Bring your big toe knuckles to touch underneath your seat, keep your knees about hip distance apart here. Six full cycles of breath.

From child's pose, reach your arms out in front of you if they aren't already, and curl your toes under, coming back to down dog. Look toward your hands and wander your feet all the way up in between them. Inhale, extend your heart forward like you did earlier—

fingertips aligning with toes, or hands on shins or a set of blocks—exhale, fold in. Inhale all the way up to standing, arms up overhead (urdhva hastasana). Then, back to tadasana, hands at your heart or alongside your body as you pause in your mountain.

We're going to string all of this together for surya namaskar A (sun salutation A).

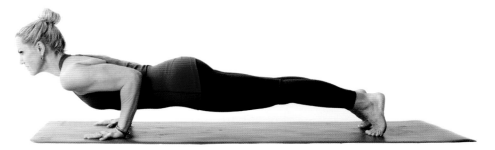

**From tadasana, inhale your arms up overhead. Exhale, swan dive forward. Inhale, gaze up, heart extending forward. Exhale, step one leg, then the other back into your plank—take in an inhale here and, with your knees down as we did earlier (or for some of you, knees off the ground this time), exhale and bend your elbows for chaturanga (low pushup).**

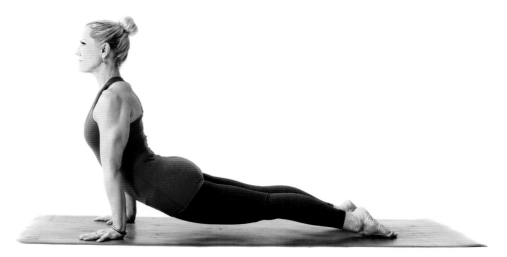

**At the end of your exhale in chaturanga, lower to your belly. Then, pull through to cobra as you inhale. Those of you more familiar with this flow might choose to glide from chaturanga into upward facing dog (urdhva mukha svanasana). This**

**means (at least in theory) that your belly stays off the floor as you roll over to the tops of your feet for your inhaling backbend. It doesn't necessarily make anything more "advanced" or better to do up dog instead of cobra, it's just a different option. As you pay close attention, one alternative may feel intuitively better to you than the other. To me that's a very sophisticated insight.**

From your cobra or up dog, curl your toes under, exhaling into down dog. You're welcome to substitute child's pose for down dog here anytime. This is your home base—a place to take inventory for a moment—to find the ABCs of your breathing and the inward turn of pratyahara. This contemplative pause is built into every sun salutation. Take six full cycles of breath in down dog or child's pose.

From here you will either walk or hop your feet between your hands (those of you in child's pose will come back to down dog first). Inhale, extend your heart forward and glance up a bit—fingertips align with your toes, or hands on your shins or blocks. Exhale and fold in, chin toward your shins. Inhale, reach all the way up (urdhva hastasana), and exhale into your mountain (tadasana) with your hands in a prayer in front of your heart or arms along your side.

That's your blueprint for surya namaskar A.

You are going to do five rounds of these sun salutations in two very different settings. Ideally you will use @OM. That way all the sequencing and timing is handled for you. Of course, you're welcome to do them on your own, but I insist that you move slowly and hold your tadasana at the beginning as well as your down dog (or child's pose) at the end of each round for six full cycles of breath. Yes, those of you who enjoy jumping back into chaturanga and hopping forward from down dog may do so (I'll be cueing that option @OM as well). If you have no idea what I mean by that, not to worry. It's another one of those alternatives you have a lifetime to explore and has little to do with what I want you to glean **On Your Mat** today.

The first time, I'd like you to do as many of the following as possible:

1. Turn on your TV loudly with the most gossipy programming you can find. Turn up the ringer on your phone, your clock radio, the pings and bells on your technology.

2. Throw your mat down carelessly—it would be perfect if an edge was curled up and the floor was slippery.

3.   Eat or drink the least light and healthy thing you can think of right before you start.

4.   Rummage through your laundry hamper and put on something dirty. A perfect choice would be something that's bound to get in your way, ride up, and require a lot of your attention.

Proceed with caution through five superslow rounds of surya namaskar A, @OM or on your own. Then we'll meet back here to continue through this chapter.

ॐ

Much like the very first tension exercise we did together earlier, did you feel that the above ingredients were incongruent to the yoga? I imagine that subtleties like your breathing, present moment, beginner's mind, paying close attention, and pratyahara (inward turn) were pretty much inaccessible. It was the flip side of your technology-free afternoon, wouldn't you say? When you create careless chaos, you generate excuses and queue yourself up for impossibility.

Wait a while before you give this a second go-around and feel free to come back to it on a different day. This time you're going to bring integrity and accountability to your mat. Before you start the sequence do this:

1.   Turn off your TV and all other sounds—well, except for **@OM**. Put your phone on "do not disturb."

2.   Thoughtfully place your mat in a room with nice light, a serene setting, and plenty of room. If there is an outside spot and the weather is agreeable, feel free to set up there.

3.   Be sure that it's been at least two hours since you've consumed anything.

4.   Wear something clean that won't distract you in any way from your practice.

5.   Sit quietly for a moment before you begin and after you've finished. Even if that's just for one minute.

Okay, either on your own or @OM, five syrupy-slow-motion rounds of surya namaskar A . . . and we will pick back up here to finish out our chapter when you're done.

ॐ

Notice how different you felt this time vs. the last time through. Right? Did you notice a connectedness to your body, breath, and focus, and the nuances of beginner's mind and inward turn?

Typically on my retreats, my students clamor into the yoga room on their first day with pieces of LA (or wherever they've come from) lodged deeply enough that they have not yet shaken them free. A familiar restlessness finds its way into our first class: there's tightness from the airplane ride and the unsteady newness of having just arrived. Some even set their cell phones next to their mat, as if they were life rafts in a sea of bothersome tranquility.

By day two, things are already different. There are pink stripes where sunblock has been missed, a few bug bites—and there has been a palpable shift. Anxiety has given way to a more relaxed, less distracted attitude that we can feel taking over the room. Our inspiriting surroundings have people bravely kicking up into arm balances they refused to do back home, and sitting still for long amounts of time in meditations they would have made excuses to miss. They've stepped outside of their routine and their norm and little by little the demands of city life (real and/or imagined) fall away.

There is nothing self-conscious about this shift. It is an organic immersion that lends itself to the universal "oneness" most spiritual practices and religions espouse. Just like you witnessed for yourself in the above exercise, when we slow down we allow ourselves to see the beauty around us, as well as within us. To quote the late Irish poet and philosopher John O'Donohue: "The human soul does not merely hunger for beauty, we feel most alive in the presence of what is beautiful—it returns us, often in fleeting but sustaining moments to our highest selves. Beauty ennobles the heart and reminds us of the infinity within us."

In yogic philosophy this infinity is called prakriti, which means "nature" and addresses the basic nature of the universe's intelligence and function. Prakriti is composed of the three gunas: sattva, rajas, and tamas. Rajas is associated with energy, ambition, and passion; tamas with inertia and darkness; and sattva with light, harmony, and goodness.

The idea is that we make our way from our self-sabotaging rajasic and tamasic tendencies and toward the balance and illumination of sattva. As my group began to surrender and merge with the beauty surrounding them, their rajasic big-city insanity became more sattvic, and they started to feel more at peace.

Daily routine can become as uninspired as that first round of mindless, harried vinyasas you took. We go through the motions and hardly remember what we're doing or where we have been. Our relationship with the concept of time has become one full of scarcity that feels fleeting, as if it were a threat. And the landscape we have created for ourselves to live in becomes more limited, linear, and constricted.

Are you navigating through your own burnout cycle? Is it your rajasic nature that has you spinning in the same circles over and over? Or are you lethargic beneath your tamasic tendencies? I've found in my own practice that understanding prakriti is a wonderful way to shift things so that I see them as opportunities to move toward sattva (illumination, and the infinity John O'Donohue was talking about). Weaving these gunas through my postures and consequently my life has helped me see that burnout can become beauty when we take the time to shine our infinite light. As Hazrat Inayat Khan said, "When we pay attention to nature's music, we find that everything on earth contributes to its harmony." Saucha is a reminder that when you're clear, quiet whispers can become the rumblings of bold possibility—in your postures and in your pursuits.

## ON YOUR OM

Saucha—the need to create an internal and external environment conducive to positive change—is now probably pretty evident when it comes to surya namaskar A, but what was tangible **On Your Mat** might feel a little bit more obscure when you climb off of it. Here too, clarity is essential, and answering the following questions will give you a better idea of what Clearing the Way looks like **On Your OM.**

I'd like you to find a notebook that you can dedicate to our cause. You're going to refer back to your entries, so you'll want to have everything in one place. Writing things down helps us see what we are living. Our words become scaffolding for our thoughts as we contemplate fresh ideas and build our new beginning. It's another way for us to pay close attention.

Find a setting that feels more like your second set of sun salutations than your tumultuous first. Take a little savasana pause. It would be terrific if you did your five-minute ABCs as part of your S.T.O.P. to S.T.A.R.T. for this exercise, creating that favorable internal and external environment. You can add to this list anytime (I do to mine), so don't feel any sort of deadline pressure.

Just begin:

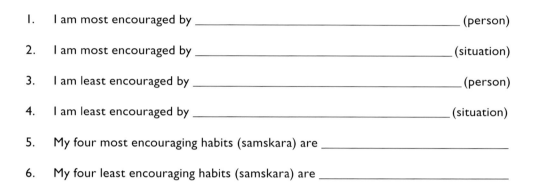

    1.   I am most encouraged by _____ (person)

    2.   I am most encouraged by _____ (situation)

    3.   I am least encouraged by _____ (person)

    4.   I am least encouraged by _____ (situation)

    5.   My four most encouraging habits (samskara) are _____

    6.   My four least encouraging habits (samskara) are _____

Now that we've jumped in and you've begun to *awaken*, isn't it fascinating to be less blinded by your internal "snow" and appreciate a new view? I mean, since our first savasana together you've been courageous enough to S.T.O.P. and S.T.A.R.T. again as a beginner. You've embraced the inside job of pratyahara. And you're witnessing ABCs as subtle building blocks for a vocabulary that communicates freedom and possibility. You've started to step out of your own way and into a new horizon.

The challenges and transitions you're experiencing on your mat during your practice give you tactile insight into life's inevitable flux. The undeniable sensations of flexibility and strength you feel first in your body translate to your mind and emotions too. Your postures are like present-moment poetry. Moving with grace through your sun salutations reminds you to do the same throughout the course of a day. Standing in your mountain (tadasana) affirms your commitment to stand into your fullest potential off your mat as well. You've awakened to how you do your yoga is how you do your life, and you are ready to *transform*.

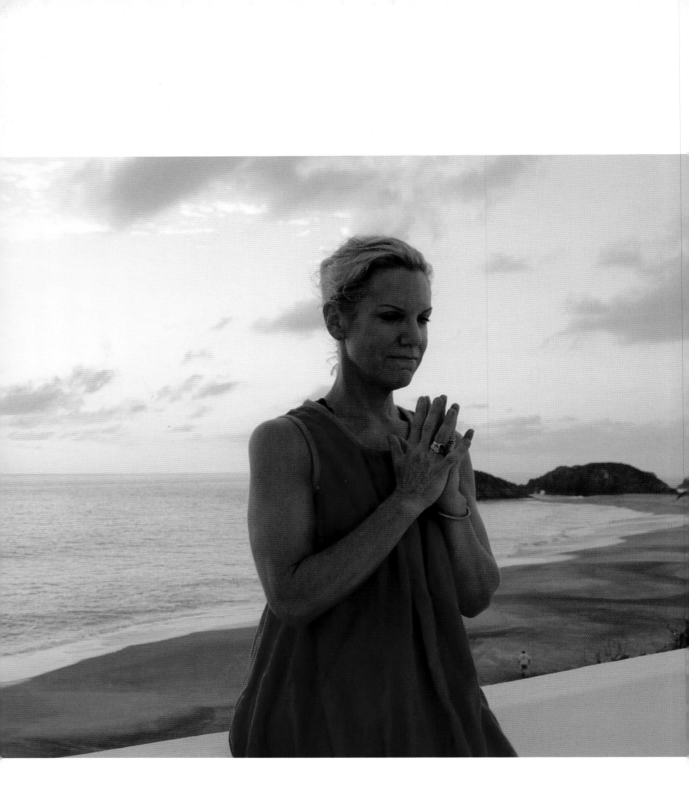

# PART II

# TRANSFORM

In this section you use your poses to go deeper, revealing what's underneath the surface. You see that in life, like in your postures, obstacles can be opportunities, practice makes progress, and that you must learn to bend and become flexible in order to move toward liberation. You transcend the limitations of comparison and competition. For example, forcing your way into a posture to the point of injury in order to compete with your neighbor will only set you back. Shifting from the perception of contest to a living laboratory allows you to learn, grow, create, and thrive. Moving from self-defeating tendencies to self-acceptance and Val-you, you focus on what your possibilities and capabilities *are* instead of *aren't* so that you can move from what you *don't* want to what you *do* want. You see that truth facilitates choices that provide vision and direction toward your full potential and most vibrant, creative life.

# 6

# What's In the Way
# Is the Way

*The impediment to action advances action. What stands in the way becomes the way.*

—MARCUS AURELIUS

**In this chapter you discover how to *transform* obstacles into opportunities.**

Much to my surprise, the first year we were married, my then brand-new husband Dom (not exactly known for his interest in the metaphysical or "spiritual") made us an appointment with Roxanna, an intuitive/psychic he'd heard about while we were on retreat in Mexico. She had us rub a bouquet of aromatherapy oils into the palms of our hands and smell them with our eyes closed for a few minutes, and then . . .

"You get frustrated," she told Dom, "and you bring it to the relationship. And Andrea tries to fix it. That is really frustrating, isn't it?"

He agreed (a bit too enthusiastically).

"You need to leave him to his frustrations," she told me. "They are positive, even though they don't seem like it at the time. They're what he needs in order to move to something better."

I think Roxanna's advice rings true for us all. We have to be allowed our seeming set-backs so that we can move through them, learn from them, and ultimately move on. To rush or to avoid this progression would be to cheat ourselves out of the gold that's being mined, and then, worst of all, we'd have to repeat the lesson. Out of the challenge comes a little shining piece to the puzzle of why. A better understanding of what we're capable of, and what we're doing here. It is our way toward meaning. Sometimes we need to get a bit lost in order to find our self.

Our yoga poses affirm that change and improvement are going to be a bit scrappy. As you and I have experienced together already, just the trials of trying to remain and breathe in a simple pose reveal that often things are not going to be as easy as we'd planned. But they just might turn out even better that way. If we take Roxanna's advice and are willing to get our hands a bit dirty, really dig deep into our personal soil and make our way down to the roots, we just might discover that when we think we've been buried, we've actually been planted.

Oh, and often it takes a little fertilizer in order for our seeds to bloom. To quote Buddhist monk and author Thich Nhat Hanh, "No mud no lotus."

It's more rewarding to do the work than it is to avoid it. We need to see balance and progress not as an isolated pose, but as a part of a larger personal pilgrimage (sadhana). When we look at things through a wider lens, we can see every fumble, challenge, and fall as an opportunity to grow. Each time we glean a little bit more wisdom to bring to our next sun salutation, handstand, or adventure.

From Patanjali's *Yoga Sutras*, pratipaksha bhavanam is the ability to look at a situation from a different perspective and turn negativity into positive action. You might say it is our beginner's mind allowing us to perceive obstacles as opportunities—to realize that what we thought was an impediment is actually hidden treasure.

When it comes to transformation, pots of gold are everywhere, often living under the heading of what we think we "suck at." Think about all the times you've found yourself saying " I suck at _____ " (fill in your favorite least-favorite pose). You suck at pigeon because your hips are tight. You suck at crow pose because you're afraid. You suck at savasana because you can't lie down for that long. And it's not just on your yoga mat. You suck at: dating, dancing, drawing, driving, deciding . . . and the problem is we allow those things we think we suck at to be where we stay stuck at.

Pratipaksha bhavanam asks us to see What's In the Way Is the Way; to contemplate and take another view; to reframe our negative perceptions and see them as opportunities; to see the blessings in our curses and to shift from buried to planted.

## ON YOUR MAT

It's that moment when we want the pose to be over that our yoga begins. That point where we go beyond the strength, flexibility, and focus we already have and begin to pioneer some new terrain. Things get uncomfortable, and all we want to do is reach for our water bottle even though we aren't thirsty, fix our hair, adjust our yoga pants—hey, we'd probably be willing to do our taxes. Just as Roxanna pointed out to Dom, brushing up against our limitations is humbling. A challenging postural moment allows us to access pratipaksha bhavanam in ways that not only further our yoga, they inform our person.

Even if you've been practicing for 5,000 years, hanging out in warrior 2 for a while gives you some serious pratipaksha bhavanam bang for your buck.

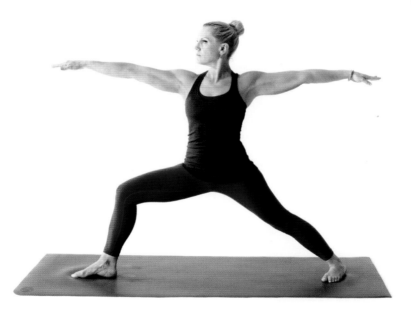

**Find tadasana in the middle of your mat facing one of its long edges. Reach your arms wide out to the side like a broad set of wings—then step your feet far enough apart that your ankles line up underneath your wrists. Bend your front knee and**

**from deep in the hip, turn your right foot to face the right short end of your mat. Shift your back heel at an angle that has your heel a bit closer to the back edge of your mat than your toes. Deepen the bend in your front knee without letting your knee go farther forward than your ankle while you continue to find tadasana in your torso. Feel free to keep your gaze where it is, or shift it toward your front hand. Warrior 2 is often explained as heel-to-arch alignment (front heel aligning with the back arch on the middle line of your mat), but every body is different, so adjust that a bit if needed. Remember as you design this posture (or any other) that you're neither chasing an outside aesthetic nor enduring sharp pain. Embracing that dull roar of progress you're feeling, however, is turning challenge into an opportunity to grow, and is pratipasha bhavanam in action.**

Imagine a racing stripe along the inside of your right thigh, elongating your inner thigh toward your front knee. Use a second energetic racing stripe running the opposite direction along the outer right thigh to draw your right hip back toward your back heel. Allow the external rotation in your right hip and the actions of your racing stripes to coerce your front knee more toward the pinky toe side of your foot instead of caving in toward your big toe.

Activate your back leg to create symmetry in your foundation. Focus on the outer edge of your back foot feeling heavy against the ground and the arch of that same foot lifting instead of collapsing. Let go of any nutty gripping in your toes, face, jaw, hands, and anywhere else you come across it. Allow the evenness of your base in the ground to guide you to an all-encompassing steadiness and surrender. With your arms outstretched, feel as though you are pressing the air down with the palms of your hands, reminding your overactive upper back and shoulder muscles to climb out of your ears and stop being so bossy. Releasing these muscles allows even the emotional drama you may be experiencing (anger and annoyance are popular) to subside, and helps you find your way to calm amid intensity.

Straighten your front leg and lower your arms to pause and rest for a moment.

 I'm not going to make you hold warrior 2 for five minutes like you did tadasana and down dog (you're welcome). But you are going to try it for two and a half minutes on each side. You can set your timer, or better yet, use @OM.

ॐ

If the physical intensity is too much, simply lower your arms for a moment or straighten that front leg (like we just did) for a second and return to the full pose when you feel ready. You're still practicing yoga—you're tuned in to your breath and your inward turn and you are listening carefully to what the sensations are telling you. In fact, I would argue that you are practicing very advanced yoga by mindfully modifying. Sometimes what appears to be stepping back is actually moving forward.

While you're holding the pose, close your eyes for a minute and feel where it's loudest to you—maybe your quadriceps screaming, or your arms yelling, or just the growl of impatience . . . oh, and your ego might step in with some suggestions. Ease back if accomplishment starts to eclipse care and consideration. When you impulsively want to leave it—don't. Stay just a little bit longer than you thought you could, using your exhales to soften the muscles and quiet your increasingly challenged mind. Keep coming back to What's In the Way Is the Way.

The treasures you uncover here are the real deal. The visceral experience you're having in warrior 2 is merely a straightforward and immediate example of the obstacles you bump up against when you're a warrior out in the world. When What's In the Way Is the Way feels elusive or murky off your mat, know that your warrior 2 here **On Your Mat** is an intuitive tune-up you can visit anytime.

Fancy poses are fine, but an ongoing relationship with deceptively simple postures is fascinating. They are a palpable reveal of who you really are in body (the frequency and way in which you sit, stand, repeat motions like reaching for your mouse or steering wheel, or carry your bag on one side), mind (where your thoughts wander off to and the stories you tell yourself), and spirit (your perceptions and emotions). Returning to these poses day after day, season after season deepens your relationship with your Self—your warrior is both a mirror and a metaphor. How we do one thing is how we do everything.

Pratipaksha bhavanam is an encouraging nudge, not an overwhelming or intimidating push. What's In the Way Is the Way turns limitations into inspiring gurus.

Now, using **@OM**, or your timer on your own, enjoy two and a half minutes on each side of your warrior 2.

## ON YOUR OM

You began to sense challenge becoming a window of opportunity in your warrior 2 both within your body (screaming quadriceps) and mind (growling impatience). Pushback becoming progress within the physical sensations of poses is immediate and concrete. But the only way to find What's In the Way Is the Way in your life is to first get clear about just exactly what it is that's in your way—to pay close attention so that you can locate the screaming quads and growling impatience of your warrior's off-your-mat odyssey too. Grab your notebook. You're familiar with a Bucket List, right? Well, you are going to write down the things in your life that are making you feel stuck right now, and we're going to refer to this as your **Stuckat List** . . . I know . . . but now it's totally stuck in your head, right? How can you forget something so unabashedly cheesy?

Think back to our first tension exercise. Remember how stuck you felt? What is it in your life that creates a similar reaction? When are you frustrated the way that Dom was in the story at the beginning of this chapter? Where do you feel buried? Where is your mud? Be thorough and know that you are welcome to add to your list anytime something occurs to you. In fact, right now you are conjuring **Stuckats** out of thin air, but when you're out in your life they will find you. Just like you've bumped up against limitations and maybe even frustrations in the postures we've done together, you will butt up against obstacles in the course of your day.

Now go for it. No editing or judging. If it enters your mind *WHAM!* it's on your page. Nobody's going to grade your work or tell you that you've passed or failed. Honesty is key. Wayne Dyer said, "If you change the way you look at things, the things you look at change." As you *transform*, you are going to change the way you look at things. First within yourself, and then in that which surrounds you . . . both **On Your Mat** and off.

# 7

# Practice Makes Progress

*Expectations are resentments*

*waiting to happen.*

—MACKLEMORE

**In this chapter you *transform* and see that expectations of perfection are a trap and perseverant practice and surrender are a means toward transformation.**

The first people I taught yoga to other than forgiving friends or giggling family members were at a very corporate gym, tucked away in a high-rise building in Century City, California. I'd gotten the job from Deb, a "step and pump" teacher I knew from my nothing's-ever-enough gym days. She was now fitness manager of Meridian Sports Club and I was the trying-too-hard-to-appear-Zen new yoga teacher.

There were exactly two participants in the class—one man and one woman. You could hear CNN blaring on the monitors outside the room along with the purring choir of cardio machines, but in our little overly air-conditioned bubble, what I could mostly hear was my fear.

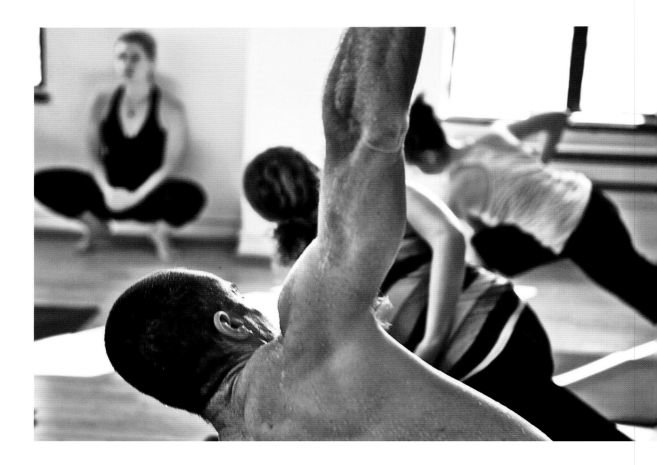

I wasn't really sure I knew what I was doing.

The man, who looked to be in his sixties, was wearing very slippery athletic socks and was dressed for a tennis court. He had a mat that would've better served him as a floatation device than something he hoped to balance inexperienced poses on. It felt like this was someone else's idea, maybe his wife's. He looked none too pleased. Instead of *namaste*, he murmured "Amen"— just in case he was exposing himself to some sort of voodoo as we began.

The female student had clearly already taken about fifteen workout classes that day. Edgy and impatient, she walked into the room talking loudly on her cell phone, and gave off a vibe of discontent before I ever opened my mouth. She lugged what looked like a suitcase of water, which was almost as big as the diamond on her finger, into the room. She also insisted on using a pair of five-pound dumbbells during the yoga practice. I was too much of a novice to utter a word about them.

As we launched into our ninety-minute class, clumsy uncertainty prevailed. At some point Slippery Socks Guy (SSG) agreed to take off his socks, and I brought him a more stable mat, but he was still not really buying it. "Take child's pose anytime you need it," I told the two of them, crawling into it myself as a guide. Meanwhile, I was the one in need of the time-out child's pose. I tried to cover my newness with botched Sanskrit and calculated sequencing. I called virabhadrasana (warrior pose) "beeradrasa" (which would have been perfect if we were at Oktoberfest), and kept confusing right from left, sometimes visiting the same side twice.

Time was moving at an insufferably slow pace. How was I supposed to fill up the entire hour and a half? I looked up at the clock, sure we were a half hour in, only to find that a mere seven minutes had gone by. I'd already rushed through three quarters of the poses I'd counted on to fill the ninety minutes at breakneck speed (including triangle no less than three times). There were eighty-three minutes in front of me, and zero ideas left in my amateur arsenal.

At minute thirteen, the woman abruptly rolled up her mat, picked up her liquid suitcase, and left without any acknowledgment. This was particularly awkward with next to no one in the room to begin with. What had I done to send her walking in a matter of minutes? I mean, she was the one using weights during yoga. What was she expecting? Was she on her way to the front desk to complain, ending my teaching career before it even started? Would SSG put his socks back on and join her?

My fear got even louder.

So there we were, SSG and me, as if on an awkward first date with nobody sure of what to say. Suddenly I remembered a Bhagavad Gita nugget: "It is undoubtedly very difficult to curb the restless mind, but it is possible by constant practice cultivating a favorable attitude in the direction of the self and by detachment from a specific outcome."

We started back at the beginning, in down dog. I explained to him that stillness was the essence of yoga and that we wanted to replace mindless movement with surrender.

So, just how did a five-thousand-year-old tradition from India, Christy Turlington, a Slippery Socked Man, the Bhagavad Gita, CNN *Headline News*, and myself all find our way into the same corporate gym?

The consensus is that yoga first arrived in the States in the late 1800s. Ralph Waldo Emerson and Henry David Thoreau were big Bhagavad Gita fans. Yogic introspection influenced Thoreau's time at Walden Pond, and in a letter he wrote in 1849 Thoreau said, "To some extent, and at rare intervals, even I am a yogi."

America initially perceived yoga as best suited for the nefarious and hedonistic. But in the 1930s its image improved a bit with the likes of Cole Porter, Charlie Chaplin, and Greta Garbo crediting it with keeping them calm. In 1946 Yogananda's *Autobiography of a Yogi* was published. "You Americans exercise your bodies and brains too much and your will power too little," he said. Interesting to note from our postmillennial vantage point.

In the 1950s, while America was engaged in the Cold War, there was a shift happening, away from conformity toward an individual determining his or her own fate. Titles like *The Power of Positive Thinking* and *Life Is Worth Living* were published. Eleanor Roosevelt admitted to enjoying headstands in the White House (but shied away from calling it yoga). The gossip rags reported that Marlon Brando, Gary Cooper, and Mae West were doing something called Hatha yoga. Marilyn Monroe said she did yoga poses to "improve her legs." Even the YWCAs and YMCAs had Hatha offerings. Many of the important Western master teachers of today like Lilias Folan and Judith Hanson Lasater took their first yoga class at their local Y.

The free love/drug culture of the 1960s cast a bit of a shadow on the mainstream acceptance of yoga (beware the hedonists . . . again).

Music producer Richard Bock introduced world-renowned sitarist Ravi Shankar to jazz musicians like John Coltrane and Indian influences found their way into Coltrane's music; George Harrison studied sitar with Shankar, and the Beatles visited Rishikesh (the "World Capitol of Yoga") in 1968 amid widespread media attention. There, on the ashram of Maharishi Mahesh Yogi, they enjoyed one of the band's most productive chapters. This prolific period included eighteen songs that were later recorded for the *White Album* and *Abbey Road*. Back in the US of A, words like *guru*, *mantra*, and *meditation* began to infiltrate the common vocabulary. It was the Age of Aquarius, of Woodstock.

In the 1970s, the likes of Ram Dass were transitioning from Harvard professors to spiritual teachers. Sri K. Pattabhi Jois, the father of Ashtanga yoga with all of its sun salutations we now hold synonymous with yoga, began to establish a Western presence. Fellow progenitor B. K. S. Iyengar did the same.

The Jane Fonda, high-impact *Flashdance* majority of the late 1970s and 1980s just didn't have the attention span for yoga. It was all about raising your heart rate and keeping it there.

Then, in the early 1990s, Dr. Dean Ornish's revelations about how yoga contributed to the prevention and even reversal of heart disease brought yoga back into the conversation in a big way. Madonna impressed everyone with her Ashtanga arms, and Sting told tales of being able to have sex all day long because of his yoga practice. All this PR shot yoga into a new stratosphere. Before you knew it—in gyms, studios, parks, even on paddle surf boards—toe-ringed, green-tea-drinking Republicans joined insatiable, yoga-gear-consuming Democrats, athletes, recovering veterans, celebrities, cancer survivors, and pretty much everyone else in downward facing dogs all across America.

When I adjusted him as I'd learned in my teacher training, his body responded to my direction. His arms began to shake as his muscles learned to open up and remain stationary. He willingly took child's pose to rest for a moment, and we had a refreshing chuckle about how such a simple pose could be so difficult.

He humbly agreed to modify his vinyasa by putting his knees down for plank (top of a pushup) and chaturanga (bent-elbowed bottom of a pushup), and then to lower all the way to the ground for a safe cobra instead of an up dog. "In cobra pose your hips and legs stay on the ground as your upper body gently arches into a backbend, in up dog everything comes off the ground except for the tops of your feet and your hands. Cobra's not as risky as up dog for your lower back." I sounded like my syllabus without needing to refer to it. I *had* retained some of its information after all!

As we moved into some of the warrior poses, I asked him to step his right foot forward between his hands. He looked at me as if he had no idea where he might find his foot or his hands and he nervously stepped his left foot forward. My earlier dyslexic faux pas left me sensitive to the fact that were I to have pointed out he'd stepped with his left and not his right, I'd only have made him more self-conscious. I was learning that sometimes you'd have to set down the rulebook and go with your gut. Even as he wobbled in the pose, we'd both become a lot steadier. As we made our way into the quieter seated poses of our cool down, I was surprised to look up and see that there was just enough time left for us to end with a five-minute savasana.

SSG and I were part of a lineage of fits and starts that these days has translated into a billion-dollar wellness industry. But in the months to come we would discover something together that exceeded any trend or media hype. SSG returned to my class every week. Through our practice together, we began to develop clarity, discipline, and a kind of faith. I was getting my footing, and so was he (especially now that he was sock-free). Fear gave way to understanding, and more and more students came and joined us.

When the holidays came around, SSG gave me a Ryuichi Sakamoto CD, and asked if I could write down "some of those poses" for him so that he could do them in his hotel room while on vacation with his family. We had inspired in each other two key components found in that earlier Bhagavad Gita quote as well as Patanjali's *Yoga Sutras*: abhyasa (persevering practice) and vairagya (surrender).

All of us stumble, especially when we're transitioning toward something new or unfamiliar. We need time and even an occasional child's pose to ease in—to S.T.O.P., S.T.A.R.T., breathe, become present, turn inward, and give ourselves internal and external support. Abhyasa and vairagya demand that we resist the trappings of instant gratification and expectation that modern society seems to promote. Like Charlie Chaplin and the other unassuming yoga-inspired who'd come before me, the abhyasa and vairagya I found at Meridian Sports Club was, in a sense, my Beatles visit to Rishikesh. It showed me I could turn humiliation into illumination. As Ralph Waldo Emerson so famously put it, "Life is a journey, not a destination." And as ongoing beginners we feel ourselves start to *transform* as we discover it's not about whether we ever grab our big toe. The prize is in the reach.

## ON YOUR MAT

**On Your Mat** you're going to assign yourself a **Possibility Pose**. It can be anything, but try to have it be something you find challenging and feel **Stuckat**. You're going to use this posture to show you where you might fall into the trappings of expectation or futility of "perfection." Here's an example from one of my workshops to give you an idea of what I mean.

Kirsten was a competitive CrossFit athlete. She declared to the group before we started our practice that full backbend (urdhva dhanurasana) was her **Possibility Pose**. She'd tried and tried to wrap her mind and her kettle-bell-swinging, Olympic-weight-slinging inflexible shoulders around urdhva, but it just seemed like something other people could do but not her. The expectation that Kirsten needed to recognize, acknowledge, and then transform was her story of urdhva impossibility. Heavy lifting came easily, but mobility was her challenge. A challenge she'd gone to great lengths to avoid making eye contact with.

As it turned out, it wasn't just about tight shoulders: urdhva was a metaphor for the tight schedule she was **Stuckat** off her mat too. Running her own CrossFit gym had her feeling boxed in (actually, in CrossFit-speak gym translates as "box"). She knew she needed to stretch outside of her box, but it was hard to wriggle free from the daily grind of responsibility she was **Stuckat**. The pliability of a backbend mirrored her need for elasticity and openness in her life.

It just so happened that Kirsten had joined nearly one hundred lululemon ambassadors and myself for a weekend summit I was leading called Dare To Be. Our workshop took place at the Wanderlust Festival in Lake Tahoe. Instantly, Kirsten's punishing WODs (workouts of the day) were replaced by Wanderlust's henna tattoos, kombucha tea, free spirit flow, and lying on the floor with stretchy-panted strangers for what seemed like forever. "I called my mom to tell her that I'd actually participated in a Courage Dance," she told our group. The freedom she was feeling from stepping outside of her norm had her wearing a halo even more spectacular than the flower-child variety available for purchase at the festival.

And her breakthrough wasn't limited to boho beatitude. In the yoga room, her dance with courage continued. Holding on to my ankles as an elevated foundation, Kirsten and I untangled **Possibility** as I carefully hoisted her up into her first precarious urdhva dhanurasana.

"Holy shit!" Kirsten exclaimed, trembling with excitement and uncertainty in her newly discovered extension. The entire room erupted with cheers. It was the chrysalis of an ongoing, daring conquest combining suppleness and strength that reached far beyond a single pose and deep into the arch of what is possible. Sometimes we have to bend over backward a little bit to see our potential.

Embracing possibility requires courage and patience, abhyasa and vairagya—not just for Kirsten, but for all of us—and it's often hidden in the folds of what we've not yet allowed ourselves to see. Your **Possibility Pose** is a tangible tool you can use alongside your **Stuckat List** to begin again, recognize what's possible (What's In the Way Is the Way), and *transform*. You'll work on this pose as a part of every yoga practice for a month, and observe yourself in the process. Think of yourself as being on safari, not rehearsing for a performance. Enjoy studying the wild animal that is your brain. Instead of chasing the end result, map your progress so that you can better understand how you arrive at it. There is no way any one of us is going to stay with something over time if we don't enjoy it. If you don't have fun with this, you won't stick with it, so have a good time. Practice Makes Progress.

I'm going to lead you toward bakasana (crow pose) as our **Possibility Pose** prototype. It's an extremely popular choice at my workshops because for many of us it represents a fair amount of fear. It also lends itself to a number of different iterations and experience levels along our way. Bakasana doesn't have to be your **Possibility Pose,** but you can use this deconstruction as a guideline for incremental progress when it comes to your own.

> **Begin by finding your way into child's pose. Your arms can reach in front of you, or you can run them alongside your body (for a refresher see photo on page 47). Adjust the width of your knees. Farther apart will give you more room to snuggle in, closer together may give you more stretch along your back body. Feel free to play with this a little. You could even sit on a cushion, pillow, or a block if you have one. And it might feel really nice to roll up a blanket or beach towel and situate it as padding between your heels and your sit bones as reinforcement for your knees as part of your set up. Placing a block under your forehead can be lovely support as well. It's all about finding a position agreeable enough for you to be still.**

We tend to think of the term "asana" as meaning posture or pose and assume it to involve physical prowess or flexibility, but it actually translates as "comfortable seat." In the Eight Limbs of Patanjali's *Yoga Sutras*, asana comes before pranayama (breath work) on purpose. We can't be agitated and restless and hope to focus on the subtle nuances of our breath. And comfortable seat is not only our physical stance—it means being comfortable sitting with ourselves psychologically too. I find this to be the juiciest, hardest, and most fruitful part of the equation.

Allow your child's pose to become a place where you can S.T.O.P. to S.T.A.R.T—where you can cultivate your breathing (pranayama) and your inward turn (pratyahara). If you opted to stay here and make this your **Possibility Pose** it wouldn't bother me one bit.

See if you can direct your breath to come in and out of your nose. Try to stay with this. If you find yourself breathing through your mouth, don't judge or condemn your mouth-breathingness and send yourself down the slippery slope of all the other things you think you can't do . . . just notice it and shift back to moving the breath in and out through your nostrils. All you can do is the best you can do. Remember, ease is essential. See if you can find the even breathing (sama vritti) from our earlier breath exercises and weave it in here. If that's going well, begin to add your ujjayi sound—the catch at the back of your throat that you can hear and feel.

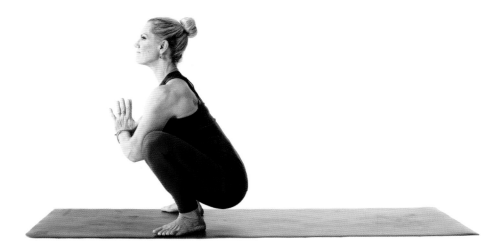

**Bakasana (crow pose) begins as a squat, and that might be where it remains. Or perhaps at some point your crow leaves the ground and takes flight. Either way, we are going to start at the beginning. Remember, we're all beginning again.**

If your hips are tight or you are feeling this a lot in your calves, shins, ankles, or lower back, you are going to want to take a generous stance. Start with hip distance, and if you need more room don't hesitate to take your feet a bit wider and perhaps angle the toes out farther than the heels. It might be helpful to sit on a block or two, or to situate them beneath your hands for more support. You also might like to take that rolled up blanket or beach towel and place it underneath your heels if they're way off the ground. There's a lot of flexibility required to squat like this, and the longer you hang out in it the louder the sensations become, so be kind. As we know from other poses we've done together thus far, just because it looks simple when we see other people do it doesn't mean it's easy when it's our turn. That's the beauty of yoga and what keeps it interesting no matter what version of the pose we're doing and no matter how many years we've been doing it.

If your squat is feeling pretty steady, bring your hands into prayer position in front of your chest. Let your elbows gently nudge your inner thighs away from one another as opposed to the knees collapsing in toward each other. This allows for a deeper stretch. Pay close attention to what you're feeling. Sharp or electrical sensations are a warning not to go so far, whereas the dull roar of something happening is progress.

Note your breath, smooth and steady through your nose. Let the inhales grow you tall in the spine and the exhales calm and root you like a truncated tadasana (mountain pose). Allow the sensations you are feeling to contribute to instead of distract you from a sense of inward turn. Get a 360-degree view of your yoga and make peace with what is instead of frantically yearning for something that isn't. Be inquisitive instead of impatient. Finding these subtleties might hold more learning potential than visiting the fully formed pose. Notice where your mind wanders off to and gently encourage it back to the project at hand. Take a good look around while you're here. You could do this version of crow all month long and glean so much fascinating information from it.

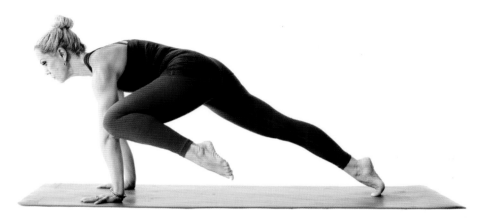

**If and when you feel ready to take this a little bit further, try this. Come into a plank (upper pushup) position. Spread your hands wide and keep them shoulder distance apart on your mat. Feel your forearms draw energetically toward one another, adding strength to your foundation. Shift your body forward enough that your shoulders are right over your wrists—this is where they'll need to live when the full pose comes into the picture. It's probably farther forward and more precarious than you are used to. Just have fun experimenting.**

Draw your low belly in toward your spine, feeling a connection deep into your core. Bring one knee to touch the outside of your arm as I'm doing in the photograph. To dial back the intensity a bit, feel free to place your back knee down on the ground and negotiate your front knee against the arm from there. In my opinion core strength has as much to do with cultivating courage and commitment as it does building muscles. Let this full spectrum of discovering your core blossom while you play here. As you repeat this over the days, weeks, or the entire month, you will get stronger and you will learn a lot about balance. Some of that's literal balance on your arms, but much of it will have to do with a larger sense of balance—one of effort and surrender. Here too notice your breath, any anxiousness or tension you are contributing, and any judgment or comparing you might be up to. Find your way back to your safari.

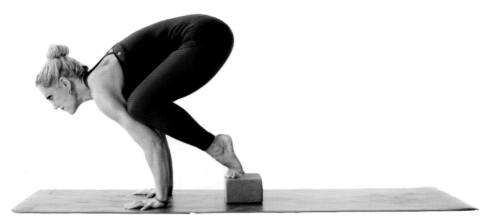

**If you're ready to give the full pose a shot, from your squat you'll crouch down to prepare for the arm balance. A fantastic way to add training wheels here is to use a block beneath your feet in your squat.**

You'll need the flexibility to keep your feet pretty close together in order for this to work. Whether from your block or from the floor, in your squatting position snuggle your knees near your armpits on the outside of your arms like you were doing one at a time in your plank. Get a feel for the pose without leaving the ground.

Gaze as far forward as you can from your perch and introduce the concept of the pose to your body and mind. Be willing to stay with this variation if that's what's most appropriate. Remember, expectation isn't invited to this party. Notice how much more comfortable you become with the idea of the arm balance just by repeating the prep in a committed, focused way over the course of a few days or weeks without trying to take on too much. What was initially foreign has made its way into your consciousness.

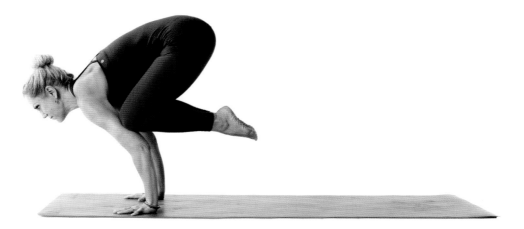

**Next, try coming up onto your toes on your block or on the floor and moving your body weight further forward with your shoulders aligning over your wrists just like we found in our plank variation. Enjoy the newness of this uncertain point of balance, and stick with that for as long as you'd like. Once you're feeling familiar with the forward shift, think about bringing just one of your feet off of your block or off the ground and start to draw that heel in toward your butt. Be calm and lighthearted as you find your way. Don't get ahead of yourself. Whether you eventually convince both your feet up by the end of the month or not, what's interesting is how you've witnessed yourself learning something new. Just keep trying, and enjoy the process.**

If you're more experienced at bakasana, you could make eka pada bakasana (single legged crow) your **Possibility Pose**. From full crow pose, try taking one of your knees off the back of your arm. Step one is to draw that knee into your chest, hovering off the ground and between your arms for a few breaths. I often explain this to be a puzzle like Pick Up Sticks but with your body. (Remember that game where you would try pulling out a stick from your stack without having the whole thing fall down?) Finding balance without the symmetry of both knees on the back of both of our arms is tricky business. Oh, and that blossoming core we were talking about will be kicked into high gear here too. I attempted this for years, so have patience. There is a fair amount of engineering that goes along with keeping your Pick Up Sticks from collapsing, and that takes time to negotiate and finesse.

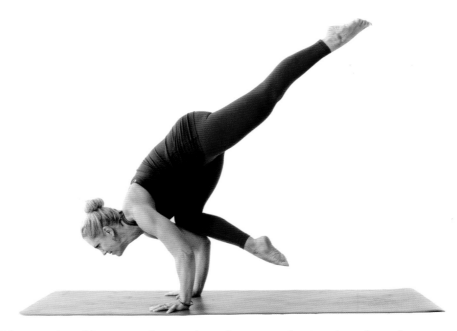

When you're able to sustain your knee into your chest and are hovering, you can start to think about extending that leg off the ground and straight back behind you like you see in the above picture. Your body will feel like a human seesaw as you dare to lean even farther forward than you have thus far so that your back leg doesn't pull you down to the ground.

A very helpful way to understand just how far forward you have to lean is the dolphin pose prep pictured below. Take a down dog on your forearms (dolphin).

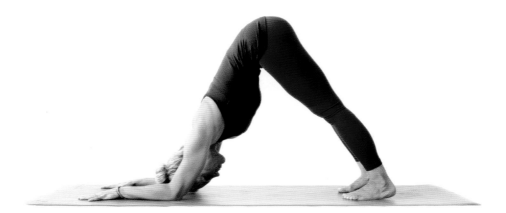

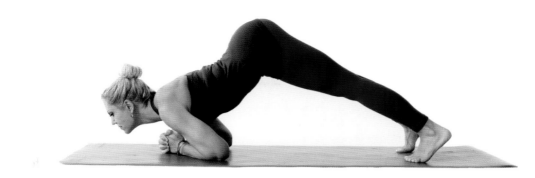

**Walk your feet in a little bit closer to your elbows and shift your body so far forward that your chin brushes the ground.**

Notice where you are in space, and then shift back into your dolphin (ugh, I know . . . easier said than done). Repeat this a few times. The prep will give you an invaluable vantage point from which to view all of these crow variations.

Still not challenging enough?

**Shoot your crow into a handstand . . .**

Think you're going to be happier once you're in a handstand? I've seen some pretty unhappy handstanders in my time. Beware of boarding the Nothing's Ever Enough train. I'm more than a little bit familiar with that ride and can spare you the detour. It's a route that will take you to Exactly Where You Didn't Want To Be and leave you looking for Even More. Just saying . . . And at the end of the day, a handstand is really just down dog with your legs up a little bit higher.

Oh, and all those times you bobble in your crow or try to get that second foot off the ground or leg to extend back behind you to no avail? They are the pot of gold. With each attempt you're deepening your understanding of yourself. Incrementally you're learning a little bit more than last time.

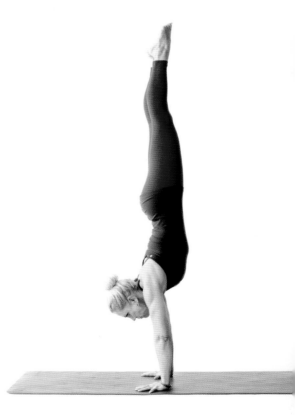

Your pose is not limited to physical accomplishment or fancy calisthenics. It is a living laboratory where you can experiment with elements like fear, balance, flexibility, patience, and commitment. You are implementing dharana (concentration) and tapas (disciplined use of our energy) in very palpable ways. Though these discoveries are happening **On Your Mat** they translate to life off your mat too, and that's really potent business. When you're truly invested in your own learning you're not threatened by someone else's process. You're inspired by your own. You're enjoying your abhyasa and vairagya safari.

Apply this quest to your own **Possibility Pose**. Allow it to become a tactile vehicle for Practice Makes Progress. There's no shortage of **Possibility Poses** out there, and yours will change and evolve as you go. Both the one you're working on now, and those you are drawn to in the future. I've had people choose anything from handstand to pigeon pose, sirsasana (headstand) to savasana. Making your way toward possibility is an expedition that takes you from blind spot to blessing—from **Stuckat** to What's In the Way Is the Way. Welcome to the jungle.

## ON YOUR OM

As I mentioned earlier, radical transformation comes in subtle shifts. Sri K. Pattabhi Jois, the father of the Ashtanga style of yoga, stated, "Do your practice and all is coming." He didn't say, "Do your practice and kurmasana (flipping your feet behind your head) is coming instantly." Nor did he promise results like millions of dollars and six-pack abs. You have to allow incremental progress to eclipse your need to accomplish the finished product or appear "perfect." Not just on your mat but off it too. Abhyasa and vairagya demand that you resist the trappings of instant gratification and impossible perfection modern society seems to promote. Think of it as R.A.T.-ing out your expectations:

R. **Recognize.** Don't be fooled, expectations are not the same as healthy intentions or goals. Expectations leave you with resentment when you don't get the result you wanted. Intentions and goals guide you without judgment in a progressive direction without attachment to a specific outcome.

A. **Acknowledge.** Acknowledge that you are experiencing expectation.

T. **Transform.** Transform your expectations into intentions—S.T.O.P., S.T.A.R.T., breathe, become present, turn inward, and allow your beginner's mind to shift you from expecting perfection to enjoying progress.

Abhyasa and vairagya are like planting your seeds and watering them every day. You wouldn't expect a seedling to grow and bear fruit overnight. Take a look at your **Stuckat List**. Choose five items on this list and ask yourself the following question:

**How did my actions contribute to this situation?**

Remember that you are not being graded or scored and that this work is for your benefit. All I ask is that you linger in the question, in the "constant practice cultivating a favorable attitude in the direction of the self" and that you not expect the "perfect" answer right this second. Remain curious as you begin the process of how to *transform* what you once viewed as an obstacle into opportunity.

Oh, and speaking of remaining curious. Are you being consistent with your "pay close attention," daily savasanas, and ABCs? Just checking. It's important that you stay on the field and not get lured back into the complacency of stuck in the stands.

# 8

# Learning to Become Bendy

*Live as if you were to die tomorrow.*

*Learn as if you were to live forever.*

—MAHATMA GANDHI

**In this chapter you see that when you Become Bendy your "mistakes" become opportunities to learn. Learning is an essential extension of your beginner's mind and a vital part of how you *transform*.**

My husband, Dom, started taking boxing classes, and wanted me to come too. So, clueless as to what I was in for, I joined him.

Terry Claybon choreographs fight scenes in movies such as *The Hurricane* and is boxing coach to stars like Denzel Washington and Matt Damon. And now here he was trying to coach me. Terry's an incredible teacher, patient but firm and all about the basics.

"You don't have to throw a single punch to be boxing," he said as we started our footwork.

It couldn't have been more different from the yoga I practice daily. Totally overthinking everything, I didn't know my left from my right. "Loosen up," Dom mouthed to me like a hopped-up Little League parent on the sidelines. That only made me more self-conscious and confused. Wait a minute, wasn't I the yoga teacher who was supposed to find calm amid intensity?

I was a disaster.

Suddenly my compassion for those brand-new to yoga was off the charts. I couldn't remember the last time I had set out to conquer something so completely unfamiliar. How was it that things that looked pretty straightforward when someone else was doing them were so hard for me to grasp?

I felt like I needed to learn how to learn.

Adele Diamond is a neuroscientist and specialist on learning. She says that we learn best by doing. "The more of you that gets involved—the body, the emotions, everything—the more you get out of it in many ways." When we have an experience of something, it's far more likely to stay with us than if we are sitting and having it told to us in a lecture. Cultivating skills and the ability to problem solve will serve us better in the long run then cramming for an exam and forgetting most of what we memorized simply to pass the test.

We glean more from being dedicated to something challenging over a period of time than we do from only participating in those things for which we exhibit insta-aptitude (oh, hi **Possibility Pose**). Modern research suggests discipline is more important than innate intelligence when it comes to our ability to learn. Having follow-through (tapas) and focus (dharana) are key. Physical activity is beneficial to brain function (another reason to do our asana). A sedentary life and unhealthy body lend themselves to poor brain health.

And, perhaps most important of all—we have to *want* to learn. That means we have to loosen our grip on a few of the things we think we know . . . sorry.

Becoming a beginner means a willingness to learn. Learning is beginner's mind and Becoming Bendy called to action. We get so attached to what we think we already know—the "right" way to do a yoga pose or practice, "our spot" in the yoga room, how our favorite venti triple-shot latte should turn out every time, how best to micromanage our daily grind—that we become unwilling to bend, even just a little. I've had students leave my classroom because they didn't get "their spot." But when we limit the ingredients, everything starts to taste the same and eventually we get burned out, uninspired, and even more inflexible. Stuck in this insipid, unoriginal loop, we find ourselves susceptible to the trappings of comparison and competition.

Becoming Bendy allows us to shift our perspective from contest or performance to laboratory experiment. When we do, we lose the competition and are no longer burdened by "success" or "failure," "good or "bad"; we're just observing and learning. Give it a test drive the next time you catch yourself comparing away on your mat, at work, in your bathing suit, or in your relationships. S.T.O.P. to put on your lab coat and S.T.A.R.T. to tinker in your laboratory instead of entering another contest. Begin to see that possibility is fluid and limitless, whereas comparison and expectation are rigid and easily broken. Feel free to test that theory under your microscope.

As we Become Bendy we also start to understand that "mistakes" are an inevitable part of learning. It's what we make of our mistakes that is key. Miles Davis said, "Do not fear mistakes. There are none." And some of history's most innovative and brilliant inventions and advancements were initially deemed mistakes by the conventional wisdom of the time. Missteps often lead to far more interesting terrain. To Become Bendy is to hang out in the ambiguity of a question long enough to enjoy the ongoing rewards of unfinished business—to be limber enough to appreciate that being a disaster in the ring is actually part of insightful discovery and growth.

Our progress is uniquely our own—not a contest with someone else. When we lose the competition, mistakes become an exciting part of what we're learning instead of a reason to feel defeated. We cannot *transform* without bending, stretching, and learning from our mistakes. Our boxing stance and our warrior poses are simply metaphors for how we step out into our lives—and there's more out there to learn than we even know.

Learning isn't about chasing achievement. It's about bending our inner control freak in new and inspiring directions. I wasn't going to boxing class to become a prizefighter. My time in the ring was more like being on safari with our **Possibility Pose**—a new opportunity to learn and expand. And at the end of the day, I was perfectly happy being one of those punchless fighters Terry mentioned—although you never know when a left hook might come in handy.

# ON YOUR MAT

Learning something new can feel like going to France with only a couple of semesters of high school French. Everything seems to be coming at you fast and furious and you can't make much sense out of it. Much as we did in our Clearing the Way chapter, we want to create conducive instead of confusing space for learning.

Let's start with a clean, clear commitment to wanting to learn. Unlike the subtext of impossible New Year's resolutions that convince us we're horrible creatures and must change into something else as soon as the ball drops, sankalpa is setting an intention with the understanding that we are perfect and whole already—even as we work toward something better.

San (connection with Source, highest Self, truth) kalpa (resolve, vow) provides an encouraging declarative platform to stand on as we Bend and learn. Don't get me wrong: it's not a gossamer excuse not to try. It's the understanding that we will get nowhere beating ourselves up and convincing ourselves we're broken and need to be fixed. Consider it an emotional S.T.O.P. to S.T.A.R.T. with the awareness, benevolence, and calm of our breathing ABCs. No one is a louder, more disruptive critic to our progress than we are until we aren't anymore.

As we learn, we are essentially creating new memories—replacing some old notions and building upon others—shifting our samskara (engrained behavior patterns). On our mat, yoga allows us to learn using a synthesis of body, mind, and spirit. We acquire skills through experience and expand on them as we draw them back up and work on them again and again. When we've previously been exposed to stimulus, even if we are not consciously aware of it, we are faster to recognize it the second time around. I reassure my newbies of this all the time. They can be totally lost in their initial class and feel like they've retained nothing. But, inevitably, when they return the second time, even if they've done no practicing in the interim, they are able to grasp the instruction and the poses faster. (Think of a couple of weeks later in France, and now you're familiar enough to manage "*où sont les toilettes?*")

As sankalpa suggests, we have to meet ourselves where we are in order to move forward. There are people who come into my classroom with the most amazing ability. They glide like swans through their standing poses and float as if levitating in mayurasana (peacock pose). Certainly there is an elegance that cannot be denied and an ease that it is hard not to lust after and compare ourselves to. They have a sheen that makes us think that life must be so much better over there than it is over here. Over here, where we reach out with our strap as if casting a fishing net, trying to wrap it around our foot and pleading with our hamstrings to let us in just a little bit. Over here, where we can hear our high school phys ed injuries and years of running on tarmac slap each other five.

Yes, aptitude is alluring, as is a colorful sunset, but the strength of the human spirit is what really steals the show. As much as we may enjoy doing them, we don't learn much from things that come easily. Daily, I watch the most unassuming practitioners create grace out of some pretty unlikely ingredients. It is less about what we may or may not have been given, and more what we make of what we've got.

In our lives, things won't always come easily, which is exactly where we'll collect the most wisdom, witness the most benefit, and enjoy the rewards of earned understanding. It's where we'll keep learning to find the lotus in the inevitable mud. Becoming Bendy is to see in an ongoing way What's In the Way Is the Way and Practice Makes Progress. It's absolutely essential that we understand our yoga as a practice, not a performance; a learning laboratory, not an audition.

A calm brain is more responsive to learning. Just as we feel a more natural state return to our muscles and emotions when we become relaxed, the same is true for our brain circuitry. You felt that happen with our tension exercise, and I'm sure you've had the experience of being so stressed out that your mind goes blank. It's what I combat every time I anticipate having to speak in front of people—don't you? But just as there are positive and negative samskara (engrained behaviors), there is "good" and "bad" stress. Actually stress itself is neutral. To a great extent it's how we wear our stress that allows it to become constructive vs. detrimental. Eustress is stress with a positive correlation— think falling in love, an exhilarating idea, or endorphin-euphoric workout. It's important to understand that we're never going to totally eliminate stress, just reshape our understanding of it and manage it.

Try this:

Lie down on your back with your one hand on your heart and one hand on your belly. Feel the rise and fall of your breath. Think of nothing other than slowing your breathing down to a fuller, richer, wider inhale and a more complete exhale. Add a beat of retention at the top before you exhale it, and a beat at the bottom when you are empty. S.T.O.P. to S.T.A.R.T. Feel the ABCs of your breathing. Give yourself a few minutes here.

With your mind now less cluttered, consider this: **setu bandha sarvangasana . . .**

Some of you will know immediately from the Sanskrit name which pose to go to, and how to arrive at it. Some of you will need for it to be translated as "bridge pose" before memory serves, and you still might be unclear about how to get into it.

Those with little or no experience of what's been requested will have to look at it and be guided into the pose with much detail, as you begin to learn and process it. If no bridge to past experience has yet been built (I couldn't help myself), there's simply not enough memory and experience to draw from. The more you practice, the more you'll remember, and you'll pull the information up sooner and faster. You'll also begin to group the information instead of it being separate bits as you build your bridge.

Before you climb further into our bridge here, it would be a great idea to take a few rounds of our sun salutations from page 42 as a warm-up. Also remember to read through this next bit to get an overview. Then return to move through it on your own or using @OM.

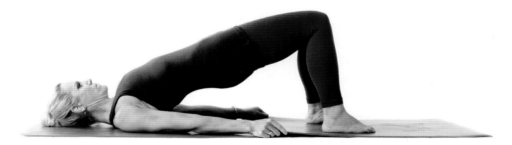

**Lying on your back, place your feet hip distance apart on your mat with your knees pointing to the sky. Clasp the side edges of your mat and encourage your shoulder blades to snuggle underneath you. Begin to lift your hips skyward with your tailbone magnetized toward your knees, creating the spacious length of tadasana in your torso instead of a compressed or compromised feeling in your lower back or neck. Try to keep your knees hip distance and pointing upward instead of flopping out to the sides like a set of ears. Energetically your shins feel like they are pulling toward your head and inspiring your chest to rise. Allow your chest to shift gently**

toward your chin, but refrain from smooshing your chin into your chest. Imagine a little egg under your chin that you don't want to crack but you also don't want to lose. Let it be the back of your head that's on your mat, and be careful not to turn side to side while you're here. Remember your interlaced cobra earlier? See if you can add that understanding of shoulder blades imprinting the spine here too. In fact you're welcome to use that interlace in this pose. Invite the calm of savasana as you breathe six full cycles of breath here in your bridge. (You will find this instruction @OM too.)

Eventually this pose becomes one remembered chunk, and you're able to add further refinement as you draw it back up. Of course along the way you'll make all sorts of fabulous "mistakes." And the best part is, once you've "mastered" the posture you're then looking to become a beginner again.

It's not just the pose you're learning about. It's you. Can you observe where you feel strong, weak, tight, flexible, confident, uncertain in the posture without comparing yourself to someone else, yourself ten years ago, or what you think is expected? Are you able to remain in the inquiry and learn something new? Can you trade in the need to be "right" or "perfect" for the opportunity to garner something insightful and furthering? Are you willing to "live the questions now," as poet Rainer Maria Rilke put it? Consider the sweet juiciness of not yet knowing (sthira) and the embrace of steady, curious study (sukham).

Becoming Bendy is consciousness, not contortionism, and this setu bandha sarvangasana backbend is a tangible bridge to fluid possibility if you allow it to be. The poses we are breaking down in these pages will be part of longer practices you do with me, with other teachers, and in innumerable situations moving forward. My hope is that when they show up in future sequences, they feel like somatic (bodily) mantras—ongoing physical reminders of the holistically significant work we're doing here together.

Be sure to spend some time with your **Possibility Pose** . . . and while I'm checking up on you, how's it going with the savasanas, five-minute morning and evening ABCs, and are you remembering to pay close attention?

# ON YOUR OM

Like you just did **On Your Mat** with bridge pose, and as you're up to with your **Possibility Pose**, you're now going to observe yourself as a unique work in progress and embrace the opportunity to learn **On Your OM** too. After all, how you do your yoga is how you do your life. You'll lose the competition and climb into your personal laboratory to take a look around. You're not prepping for a pageant or pretending to be a prizefighter—you're investigating and harvesting new morsels of self-awareness.

I totally get that self-exploration can feel a bit exposed, like those wobbly moments in a headstand when upside down needs to become right side up and we have to muster the courage to embrace the process no matter how susceptible to an embarrassing flail we might feel. Personally I've tumbled many times, certainly out of my headstand, but ultimately into a new headspace. Stumbles are an inevitable aspect of learning—and I assure you, I too am still learning.

For this next exercise it's essential to Become Bendy and to remember sankalpa. You are perfect and whole—you're just also open to new information from which to grow. Think of it as building upon the saucha (clarity) you encouraged back in chapter 5. This is an experiment, and experimenting is another way to enhance our learning.

Write down the answers to the following conversation with yourself:

1.  My best attributes are _____.

2.  I feel powerful when _____.

3.  I am most inspired when_____.

4.  I feel weak when _____.

5.  What I wish for most right now is _____;

    in five years is _____; over my lifetime is _____.

I want you to be honest with your answers. This work is for you, not for anyone else's eyeballs unless you see fit. It's part of understanding the difference between practice and performance. Consider it the wobbly headstand of your personal development, and every single one of us feels a little bit vulnerable when it's our turn to do it. Even here be on safari a bit as you take note. Which of the questions was the most uncomfortable for you to answer? Why? Take your time. Come back to this as often as you'd like. We'll be returning to these responses as part of our progression. I've kept my answers to these questions from years ago and it is fascinating to map the ways things have shifted. I can't wait to hear what comes up for you.

# 9

# Val-you and Truth

*The truth will set you free,*

*but first it will piss you off.*

—GLORIA STEINEM

**In this chapter you discover Val-you as your recipe to *transform* self-defeating inner voice into self-acceptance, making the most of what you *are* instead of remaining stuck behind what you *aren't*. And you learn to embrace truth as a compass that points you toward progress.**

"I've been practicing with you for six years and I still can't touch my toes," one of my students stated. There was an expectation that things should take a certain amount of time and that without that validation her yoga practice had less value. But touching her toes wasn't the only thing that had missed its deadline and confirmed her theory that she was damaged goods . . . why had she not met the right man by now? Why did she only date jerks that ended up breaking her heart? "What's wrong with me?" she asked.

I think we've all discounted ourselves into the self-esteem bargain basement from time to time. I know I have. But we can't assume that touching our toes or the right guy showing up will give us value. We have to reach in and find Val-you for ourselves.

Val-you is self-respect.

Val-you means stop groveling to attain what we think we *aren't*, and get to work on what we *are*.

Val-you is the opposite of self-pity.

Val-you is the accountability it takes to follow our ultimate, and dare I say divine, path.

Like finding balance in a pose, it takes resilience and commitment to learn from a teeter and to get back up when we fall. Our Val-you will be challenged, which will present opportunities for us to Become Bendy and consequently empowered in new and important ways.

For example, awhile back I got a call from a director for a fitness-oriented yoga DVD project. When I went to meet her she greeted me at her front door in a paisley purple housedress, large black-rimmed glasses, and was just the kind of New Yorker I appreciate. She began with glowing praise for my experience and legitimacy. Then suddenly threw things into reverse with: "Your hair . . . it's a problem. We'd need to do extensions. And you have an edge we need to soften. I noticed you have a pinched look on your face in some of your online classes. We'd have to teach you how to smile all the time. You'll be in pastels—none of this black you're wearing, and you'll need to lose five to eight pounds, especially in this area [she gestured to my hips] so you'd really have to work it."

Suddenly I was that tubby Dorothy Hamill–haircut gymnast thrown out of the Central Park bathroom all over again.

I anticipated the weight comment, but it was losing the rest of me that had me concerned. I envisioned the DVD cover with me, an unrecognizable mermaid sporting a creepy ethereal grin in front of an ocean backdrop in the bargain bin at Costco, marked down for the third time.

When I called my friend to tell her, a rabid "f*#@ them" canister exploded. I could feel how easy it would be to leap into the lather with her and lick my wounds. But this DVD company was not the onerous monster she was suggesting. In fact, their list of teachers is rife with integrity. They're simply trying to sell units in a marketplace that's oversaturated and becoming obsolete in a slew of online options. And they believe they have a tried-and-true recipe that works. "The one time we put a short-haired woman on the cover it didn't sell."

Once I was able to step away and get a breath, the yogic tenet *satya* hit me like a sonic boom. Satya speaks to truth and honesty, but has an element of personal accountability to it as well. I mean, I'd looked at the DVD company's material and seen their pastel playground. It would be delusional to think there wouldn't be discussion about my looks and style as I wandered in to play on it.

In these pages you and I are experiencing that yoga insists we spend time in the trenches where the lighting is not always so flattering. In my opinion, real beauty has more to do with imperfections than it does a manufactured image. We are beautiful because we are so exquisitely flawed. And if beauty is in the eye of the beholder, then when we cultivate an eye for Val-you and Truth it allows us to see that there is radiance everywhere, even in the darkest corners and toughest of times.

Satya (commitment to truthfulness) is our wake-up call to grow up, get over it, and stop taking everything personally. We pay a price for fanning the flames of misunderstanding, insult, and deceit that gets us further from, not closer to, what is honest, progressive, and real. In a quote later made famous by Jon Kabat-Zinn, Swami Satchidananda said, "You can't stop the waves, but you can learn how to surf!" Satya is the spiritual surfboard we need to save us from the undertow of fear and judgment. It brings us back to the shores of our beginner's mind, What's In the Way Is the Way, and Practice Makes Progress.

Val-you doesn't mean we have to be everything for everyone all the time, nor does it mean that everyone is going to like us all the time. It means we need to invite and be accountable for value in our lives at all times.

As we become liable for our own Val-you we find that the steadiness and sweetness of sthira sukham and the honesty and accountability of satya are the next steps in getting past **Stuckat**, and the antidote for bargain basement self-esteem.

# ON YOUR MAT

Have you ever said something like "spill your guts," "I need to find the guts to_____," or "I have a gut feeling?"

I believe our gut is where Val-you and Truth reside.

"Core work" conjures images of billboards and infomercials with glistening washboard midriffs. My definition of core work is the opposite of merely chasing an outside aesthetic. It's the physical opportunity to get to the core of who you are and a gut sense of your Val-you. It's a corporal way to move from superficial instability to deep potency and purpose in your muscles and in your mind. In fact, you might say core work provides infrastructure for enough courage, conviction, and commitment to stand up on your satya surfboard.

Lying on your back, knees bent, feet hip distance, place one hand on your upper and one hand on your lower belly. S.T.O.P. to S.T.A.R.T. Witness your breath rise and fall as it becomes longer, smoother, and wider. Try to narrow it down to just through your nose, and play with the texture of ujjayi, allowing it to scrape across the back of your throat and create a sound like the wind or the ocean. See if you can stay with this ujjayi breathing throughout the following sequence. Your hands are now located at your epicenter—your cylindrical midline—your auspicious axis. We're going to use this as a tactile tool and a means to experience your power source anatomically, energetically, and even emotionally. (Read through below and then give it a go on your own or use @OM.)

ॐ

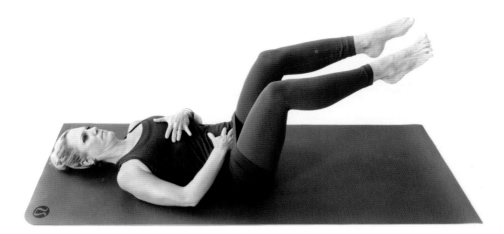

**Stay here lying down, with the back of your head solidly on the ground. Lift up your feet and bring your shins parallel to the floor. Then shift your knees a little bit further forward so that they are situated slightly in front of vertical to your hips.**

Notice muscles in your core as they work underneath your hands to stabilize your lifted legs. If you play with this dance of shins, not dropping lower than parallel and thighbones adventuring a whisper farther from your chest, you'll gather more and more core intel.

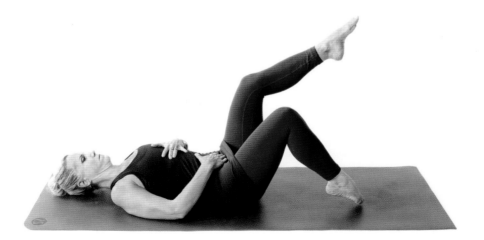

**Now bend your right knee deeply and lower your right toes down so that they just flirt with touching the ground.**

Then bring those hovering right toes a few inches forward, approximately two feet away from your right sit bone so you really feel some goodness percolating under your hands as your core engages . . . Stay here and breathe. Oops, keep your head down . . . it's so tempting to struggle in the shoulders and neck, isn't it? Stay for three to six full cycles of breath, then bring that right shin back up to align with the left. Next, lower your left toes to hover above the ground. Head stays down, toes sneak farther forward, and you let this side simmer for three to six full cycles of ujjayi breath. Then bring your left shin up to meet your right again.

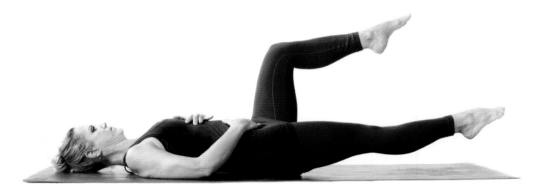

**One slightly spicier option is to scrub that hovering toe forward, maybe even to where your leg extends straight out in front of you a few inches off the ground.**

Pause for a beat or two, then gradually, as if moving through water, bend that knee and bring your hovering toe back toward your sit bone, and then bring your right leg up so that the shins are parallel again. Think of this as you take the slow, scenic route, not creating postural panic as you go. Do the same on your left side.

Ultimately you will do ten rounds of the variation that works best for you side-to-side. Meet yourself where you are and just do as many as you can today, then look forward to building on that. Practice Makes Progress. (Remember, audio guidance for this can be found @OM.)

When you've finished your ten rounds (or however many you managed), pause with your feet flat on your mat and invite the calm of a savasana, recalibrating for a moment. You're going to do that again. I'm suggesting another ten rounds, but you'll do what you can.

If you're straining in the neck or feeling this manifest as pain in your lower back, those are not sensations to endure. They're letting you know you've reached your max for today.

After your second round of ten, place your feet back on your mat and enjoy at least one full minute of simply breathing into your ABCs with your hands remaining on your upper and lower belly. Feel how many of the muscles helping you to breathe are the same as those you were working during your toe hovering just now. Hmmm. That would suggest that a stronger core lends itself to more productive and oxygenating breathing too. I bet that would contribute incredible endurance and stability to your mountain and warrior . . . not to mention be helpful as you find the guts to _____ (ask him/her out, present your idea at the meeting, show someone the writing you're working on, the painting you've been doing, your photography). Right?

Remain on your back. Reach your arms overhead on the floor, shoulder distance apart, palms facing one another. Flex into your heels as if you were standing in tadasana on an imaginary wall in front of you. Lengthen your arms and legs in opposite directions so strongly that you can feel central muscles engaging. Note that your core is actually 360 degrees—that the cylindrical midline is your side and back body as well as your front body.

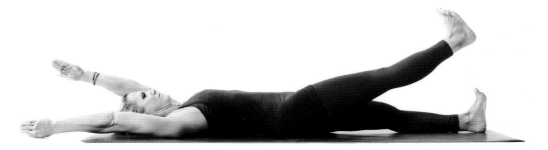

**Grow so long in your right leg that it begins to lift up off the floor. Do the same with your left arm and feel it float off your mat, leaving the back of your head on the ground.**

Stay for three to six cycles of breath. Then switch sides. Play with a couple of these on each side.

Then, keeping your arms overhead, hook your thumbs and energize them as if you were trying to pull them apart. If your lower back is tender, take this overhead arm position out of the equation. Stay lying down and just bend your knees and put your feet on the floor for a moment so you can lift your hips up, slide your hands beneath your butt, and sit on them instead. You can then straighten your legs out along the floor again, or keep your knees bent for the next part if need be. Now see if you can inspire both legs to float off the ground at the same time, the way you were doing one at a time a moment ago, whether that's seated on your hands or thumbs hooked and arms resting on the ground overhead.

If someone were to walk into the room, they might look at you and think that you were doing a very stiff savasana. If they joined you, however, they'd soon realize that this may appear unassuming, but when you're the one doing it, it's no joke. This needs to be a two-way conversation when it comes to the sensations you are feeling. Be sure that you pay close attention so that you can hear if things are starting to become too much. Stay for three to six cycles of breath, then release. Remember to keep your head down, and think tadasana through the torso.

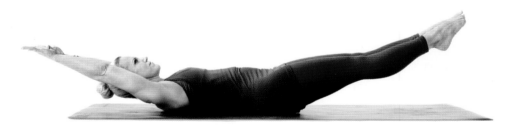

**This first variation is probably plenty. But if you want a little extra gusto, in addition to elevating your legs, lift your arms off the ground right alongside your ears. Maybe even allow the back of your head and your shoulder blades to float off your mat too. Be sure this is creating zero strain and pain—in particular in the lower back and neck—just the feeling of guts getting gutsy. I'm going to suggest five rounds of three to six cycles of breath here too. If you feel compelled to do more, be my guest. If fewer need to happen today, fabulous—you'll be beginning again and again, remember? Give yourself at least a full minute of recovery. With your knees bent, hands on your upper and lower belly, pause to appreciate your breath, an element of ease, and a return to equilibrium.**

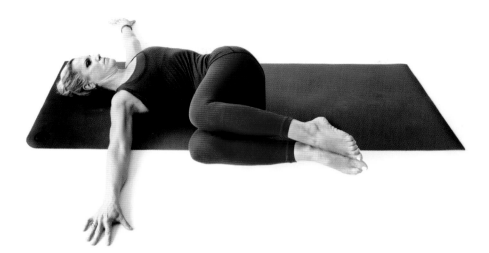

**Then, still on your back, bend your knees into your chest and take your arms out to the side, palms facing up or down. As if taking a supine twist, start to drop your legs over to the right, but stop and suspend your knees a few inches above the ground (jathara parivartanasana).**

Encourage your knees to reach increasingly toward your right shoulder and elbow, as your belly and chest twist the opposite direction (to the left). Stay for three to six cycles of breath. Carefully bring your knees back to center. Say hello to your oblique abdominal muscles in the side waist. Then glide your knees over to the left side and let them hover a few inches above the ground. Keep them the direction of your left shoulder as your chest and torso revolve to the right. Jathara parivartanasana actually means, "belly turning (or churning) pose," which I find to be quite accurate, don't you?

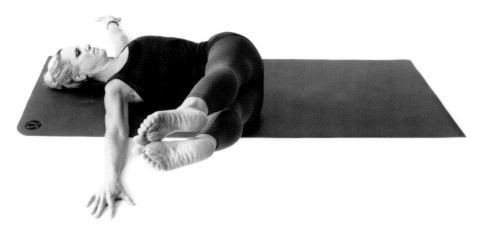

**You'll attempt ten rounds, or whatever number works for you, holding for three to six breath cycles on the right and then on the left side-to-side. Modifications and breaks are always encouraged. If you really want to add some cayenne, try straightening your legs out to the side. I usually bend my knees to return to center and then straighten them again when I get to the other side just to be sure my low back is okay in the transition.**

Enjoy a mini-savasana for a full minute when you're done. You may want to let your feet be as wide as your mat and your knees gently rest against each other to widen and support your lower back nicely. Think knock-kneed savasana to counterbalance the intensity.

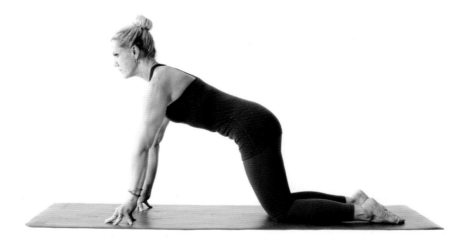

**Now climb onto your hands and knees as if preparing for Cat/Cow. Stay here and come onto your fingertips.**

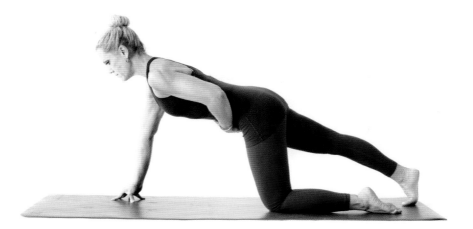

Notice how you have to become buoyant in the torso and strong in the legs in order to endure remaining on your fingertips. Take your left hand onto your low belly, kind of like you were doing on your back a few moments ago, but with only one hand. Feel a light lift of the low abdomen toward the spine (uddiyana bandha), even as you continue to breathe deeply—ideally through the nose and not through the mouth. Keep your hand on your lower abs and extend your right leg out behind you as if it were a leg in a plank.

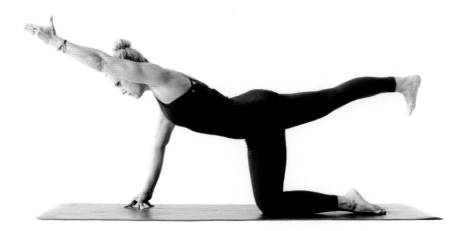

Feel the ab muscles under your left hand working toward core stability. Either keep your hand there, or take your left arm out in front of you, pinky side of the hand down and biceps aligning with the ears—almost as if you were reaching out to shake someone's hand. Now, see if you can lift your right foot one foot off the ground, but not so high it lands in your low back . . . still on your fingertips?

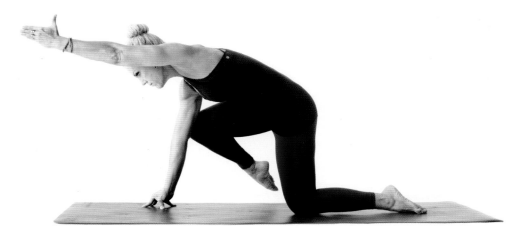

**For even more intensity (not that you need it) bring your right knee to touch your right upper arm much like you may have done in your crow pose prep on page 73. Stay light on the tips of your right fingers and feel as though you've still got a hand on your low belly (maybe you still do). Try to remain here for six cycles of breath, truly witnessing the power of your center.**

Release your first side, shake out your hands, then come back to your hands and knees on your fingertips and do the same thing on the second side. Bring your right hand to your belly. Extend the left leg behind you as if it were performing plank pose. Keep your hand on your abs, or reach the right arm out in front of you and see if you can coerce your left leg to lift just an inch off your mat. Oops, stay on your left fingertips. Oh, I know . . . Possibly bring your left knee to brush up against your left triceps (upper arm). (@**OM** will happily walk you through this sequence too.)

When you've finished both sides of fingertip fun, sit comfortably for a few moments and enjoy your connection to your center. Be sure to spend some time with your **Possibility Pose**. Then find your way to a finishing savasana. Again, rest your hands on your belly. Note it as a nucleus of confidence, a power center that reaches beyond your muscles and brings you to the core of your being even as you soften and let go. Know that you've got the guts for Val-you and Truth. Remain in savasana for five full minutes.

# ON YOUR OM

In the yogic texts, satya is described as "the truth which equals love." It implies enlightenment by way of acceptance. It is in many ways the yogic way of pointing to self-love. When we celebrate who we are and stop trying to be someone we are not, we start to brush up against things like joy and fulfillment. Few things are more attractive.

In chapter 5 you got clear about what an internal and external environment conducive to positive change looks like for you. In the previous chapter you were willing to Become Bendy enough to learn some pretty revealing nuggets about yourself. We're going to build on both of those exercises.

Since you don't live sequestered in an isolated cave in the Himalayas, there will be input and feedback in your life from outside sources and from other people. Val-you and Truth allow you to interpret this as constructive vs. destructive—encouraging vs. discouraging to your transformation. You're going to find a minimum of three friends or family members and have them answer some of the questions you did in the previous chapter. You can have them write down their answers, meet in person, or talk over the phone. All I ask is that you really do this.

1. What do you see as my best attributes?

2. When do I become powerful?

3. When do I become weak?

4. When am I most inspired?

5. What do you wish most for me right now? In five years? In my lifetime?

You will look at their responses next to yours as a remarkable window into Val-you and Truth. These insights are going to help you *transform* your **Stuckat List** into a passport to **Close to OM**.

# 10

# Choices

*The possibilities are numerous once we decide to act and not react.*

—GEORGE BERNARD SHAW

**In this chapter you see that pausing to respond instead of react is impera-tive to *transform* mindless into mindful so you can make choices that lead you Close to OM.**

Nosara is a tiny town on the Pacific coast of Costa Rica. It's a utopia for ex-pats, espe-cially those from the U.S. and Canada. On retreat there one year the importance of taking an introspective moment before we take action became dramatically apparent.

While I slept, some in my group decided it sounded like fun to go to the bullfight at the local rodeo. There they discovered a Nosara tradition wherein people (other than expe-rienced matadors) enter the bullring and stay there even after the agitated bull has been released. Mind you, this isn't something the locals feel compelled to do. It's reserved mostly for the idiot drunken tourists. So, fitting the profile, the men in my group were the first in the ring.

A widely viewed You Tube video entitled "NOSARA BULLFIGHT GRINGO LOSES" is a record of what happened next. As the angry bull careens around the ring, you can see some of my terrified idiots running for their lives, beer bottles still in hand. Then someone is violently gored by the bull . . . repeatedly. The rag doll of a man is dragged out of the ring seemingly lifeless. By some miracle, it was not one of my tribe, but the rumors of the gored man's condition followed us throughout our retreat week. For about three days the reports had him dead . . . and then alive again. Months later we would see pictures of him on the Nosara Facebook page with enormous stitched-up scars where he'd been skewered navel to neck—a smile on his face and cocktail in hand. (In case you're concerned, the bulls are not harmed at Nosara bullfights . . . just the tourists.)

In order to make mindful vs. mindless choices, we need to pause, get clear, and find viveka (discriminative discernment—aka, the antithesis of impulsive, intoxicated bozos in a bullring). Viveka lands for me viscerally if I think of it as Go to the Rodeo but Don't Get Into the Bullring. After all, bullrings come in myriad forms: taking a breath before we fire off that F-you e-mail to our boss or coworker in the heat of the moment, down that whole pint of Ben and Jerry's, fling ourselves into our deepest backbend without a warm-up, or head to the bar instead of the cardio barre class we meant to go to—any number of negligent knee jerks we end up regretting that could have been avoided with a little thoughtful stopover. Skillful awareness around the choices we make creates a shift from reaction to response.

## ON YOUR MAT

Yoga and meditation guide us to use deep, focused breaths to help us get past the things that threaten to overwhelm and deceive us—I can't be expected to do everything, what if I lose my job, what if he/she doesn't love me, what if my editor doesn't like this draft . . . As a result life feels less debilitating and more manageable.

Remember the stress response? That reaction that's often referred to as "fight or flight"? Unfortunately, in our age of constant communication, stress triggers are everywhere—we're overloaded with new stimuli and new challenges. (Ever instantly return a text to get it off your chest, only to look up and find that you've missed your stop or your flight and are even more stressed out than before?) We can see it with our computers when they're overtaxed and malfunctioning—the same is true of us. For our bodies and minds, chronic stress is like never logging off, pumping hormones and nerve chemicals longer and stronger than needed. Our relaxation response is our way of refreshing our internal screen. As you know, from our very first tension exercise together and the savasanas and ABCs you're practicing, a S.T.O.P. to S.T.A.R.T. pause helps to slow your heart rate, calm your body, and clear your mind. This allows you to make choices that come from mindful response instead of a stressed-out mindless reaction. Even if that's as simple as choosing to leave the house with enough time to pay close attention instead of panic about punctuality, protocol, or parking.

Can yoga encourage us to make more thoughtful choices?

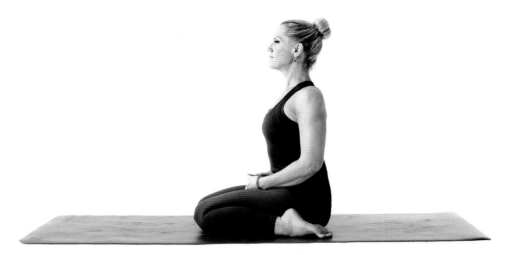

**Let's take that virasana as an example. Sitting between our heels with our knees close together and encouraging our sit bones to settle onto our mat is potentially very intense business for your knees and ankles. Virasana is "hero's pose" and out of the gate you have a number of choices to make as you build your virasana, the first being, don't try to be too much of a hero.**

Some days my Marcum knees scream as if a bull were chasing them if I try to get my sit bones onto the ground instead of onto a prop. Knees are delicate, complicated creatures with an elaborate network of finicky ligaments, tendons, and nerves. The muscles you are stretching in this pose are the motors that move the bones that meet at this vulnerable joint. When we walk, our knee supports about one and a half times our body weight; add stairs it's 3 to 4 times, squats and even warrior poses about 8 times . . . poor little things.

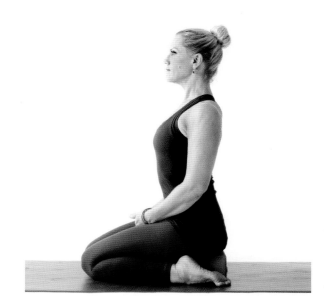

For some of us it's the feet and ankles that feel like they're being gored in this pose. You want to keep your feet aligned with your shins and avoid turning them out to the sides arch side down. Props are highly recommended. I often sit on a block or folded blanket for this pose.

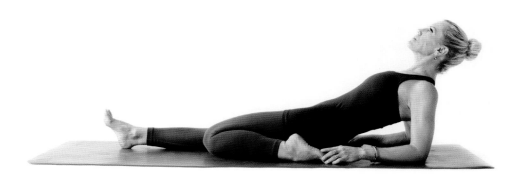

You can also do this one leg at a time to investigate safely. Straighten one leg out in front of you, flexing the toes to the sky. Cautiously bend your other leg back like a hurdler's stretch. If this is tough, slide a blanket or folded towel under your sit bones to elevate and give more space to your bent knee. Check the angle of that foot as mentioned above, and be sure to have your knees close to each other here too. Place your hands on the ground behind you and maybe even ease your way onto your forearms. Be careful not to manipulate your torso to one side or the other. Lean straight back until the sensations begin to speak to you. Go slowly, and pay attention to where you're feeling the intensity. Back off if it feels like too much on your bent knee. You'll repeat this on the second side.

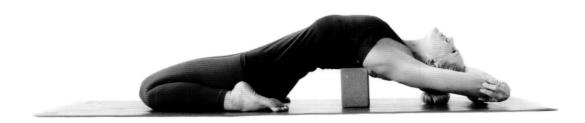

**If you're sitting comfortably on the ground without a prop underneath your seat, you might choose to lean back onto your forearms with both knees bent. Easy now. You don't want to bite off more than you can chew. Like your knees, your lower back needs special consideration. Your pelvis, hips, and lower back are highly innervated (think highway of nerves), something you want to be conscious of as you situate yourself. On those days when it feels right, I occasionally take supta virasana. I lean back and use a block underneath my shoulder blades, then take my arms overhead and clasp opposite elbows as you can see in the picture above. Sometimes a second block under my head feels great, other times the floor is where it wants to rest. Believe it or not there are people who like to lie all the way down on their back here without any blocks. When it comes to variations of virasana there's a lid for every pot—you just don't want to force a lid that doesn't fit and have your pot boil over.**

Enjoy the simplicity and intelligence of constructing a therapeutic stretch for the quadriceps muscles in the front of your leg. These muscles shorten up from sitting, walking, and driving, and when they do, that can create or contribute to knee concerns, back and hip flexor pain, and other detrimental posture issues. It's imperative to work gradually, not to use force, and to avoid sharp pain. Who cares about appearing to be a pretzel when you can feel the safe, certain liberation of the more basic variation? It doesn't have to be über-bendy, and frankly for most of us it's not. Excessive is not impressive. Modifying or using props is kind of like having the sense to switch from beer to water before we do something foolish at the rodeo—whether that's for a lifetime or just for now. Healthy choices are those we never regret, and whether you're a new practitioner or well-seasoned, "good yoga" is yoga that feels good today *and* tomorrow. Plus, when it comes to being a hero, if we can't take care of our self, we'll never be able to save anyone else.

Life itself is a fantastic rodeo. We don't want to miss out on it because we're pinned beneath the bull#%$ of our unfortunate choices. If we allow our yoga to guide us toward viveka and response, and away from impulse and reaction, we will make informed choices we can maintain. Remember, often stepping back is what moves us forward.

You're going to choose a variation of virasana to hang out in for five minutes. Pay close attention to the choices you make when it comes to modifications and why. Could there be a bit more knee-jerk bullring infiltrating your decision making than you realized? Is your ego smarting a little? Can you decide to back off and deconstruct it a bit? Make sure you're not reacting to my request by setting yourself up for guaranteed torture. Stay curious in your laboratory instead of chasing an extreme. S.T.O.P. to S.T.A.R.T.—get clear and present. Finesse tadasana in your torso, and find the ease of savasana in your chosen variation. Meet yourself where you are. Set your timer or use @OM. Then—for five minutes—Go to the Rodeo but Don't Get Into the Bullring.

Find your way out carefully once your five minutes are up. I would recommend a slow, gentle trip to down dog too. Maybe even a careful sun salutation A or two. Be sure to spend time with your **Possibility Pose** (make certain you're warmed up enough before attempting it). Are you able to enjoy the rodeo without slipping into impatient bullring reactions with that posture too? How about with your daily savasanas, morning and evening ABCs, and "pay close attention"?

To end this practice, take a five-minute savasana. Enjoy the rodeo of rich relaxation for the full five minutes here without succumbing to the bullring of "I don't have time" or "I'll do it later."

## ON YOUR OM

Building upon the respite of S.T.O.P. to S.T.A.R.T. allows you to move from involuntary impulse to mindful response, where you can use the transformational tools you're acquiring to make better choices. It gives you room to be present and turn what your beginner's mind is learning into dynamic, incredible potentials. You've been taking time to do your savasana S.T.O.P. to S.T.A.R.Ts and breathe your ABCs every day, now you'll expand upon those and develop a seated (sometimes called formal) meditation practice to create even more insightful space. Allow me to arm you with a couple of gems before you dive in. Meditation can seem intimidating and these two quotes get my meditation wig on straight every time:

*"My mind is like a bad neighborhood. I try not to go into it alone."*
—ANNE LAMOTT

Anne's pointing out what you've been dipping your toe into throughout this book and with your practices. Left to our own devices, most of us don't want to confront ourselves. People go to great lengths to dodge such confrontations and contemplation. Ah, but not you! Not any more! You've reached the leg of our journey where you can embrace What's In the Way Is the Way, Practice Makes Progress, Learning to Become Bendy, and Val-you and Truth as essential aspects of your transformation—even when it feels like you might be careening into a sketchy neighborhood.

*"If you're alone in the kitchen and you drop the roast, pick it up and put it back on the plate . . . no one will know."*
—JULIA CHILD

What Julia Child is saying is that while you're meditating, your mind is going to wander. It just is. And when it does you simply put the roast back on the plate. Actually, the act of bringing your mind back is like strengthening muscles in your mind. You are quite literally changing your mind by creating brain synapses and new neural pathways. The world of neuroscience refers to this as neuroplasticity.

Find a comfortable place to sit (which may or may not be on your mat). You can use cushions or pillows or opt for a chair with a straight back on it so that you can lean back for support but still remain upright. Some place where you aren't squirming with sensations and can remain still for a slightly longer sit than we've done together so far. You might even lie on the floor. You're going to be here for ten minutes. You can definitely build on this amount of time as you become more familiar with meditation. I have a steady twenty-minute practice at least once a day. Many people dedicate an hour or even longer. The most important part is your consistency. Don't confuse a novelty long sit followed by months of nothing as skillful integration of meditation into your life. You will find your sit fit as you go. You just have to actually keep sitting. I'd like you to start to add one minute each week to your daily ABCs. That can be an additional minute to both the morning and evening or just to one. See if you can work your way up to at least one ten-minute sit each day.

Begin by simply becoming aware of your breathing. If it's helpful, rest your hands on your chest or your belly to feel it rise and fall. Let it become slower, richer, wider, deeper, and feel a gentle pause at the top when you're full and at the bottom when you're empty. There is no rush, nowhere else you need to be, nothing else you need to do. Now simply follow the sounds inside and outside the room (or wherever you are) without commentary or creating stories around them. Sounds pull you into the present moment and out of the stories and thoughts that make their way across your path. Just listen and breathe. Super simple. Not necessarily easy. Oh, and enjoy putting the roast back on the plate . . . because I guarantee you will. Use your timer or **@OM**. Ten minutes. You can do it. Go.

ॐ

A contemplative pause is imperative for us to move from reaction to response so that we can make better choices, stay out of the bullring, and get past **Stuckat**. It gives us room to turn what we are learning into a compassionate mosaic of incredible potentials. Returning to the clarity of the present moment will allow you to begin again and make mindful vs. mindless choices **On Your Mat** and **On Your OM** that lead you to the creative space of our next chapter.

# 11

# Creating Space Is Creative Space

*Be brave enough to live life creatively.*

*The creative place where no one*

*else has ever been.*

—ALAN ALDA

**In this chapter you courageously and creatively *transform* what you've been learning into the symphony of your life.**

Getting clarity around our choices is like cleaning our windshield and suddenly seeing an encouraging landscape in front of us. Creative space is the territory between stimuli and response that acts as a contemplative greenhouse for the seeds of what we're learning to mature into blossoming intelligence. Creativity stems from investigating ideas. Creative space means living into the fluidity of possibility and having more experiences to draw from. To quote a *Wired* interview with Steve Jobs, creative people are "able to connect experiences they've had to synthesize new things. And the reason they are able to do that is that they've had more experience or they have thought more about their experiences than other people."

Integrating beginner's mind, Val-you, Practice Makes Progress, and Go to the Rodeo but Don't Get Into the Bullring is fertile ground for budding imagination and innovation. Creative space is where we manifest discoveries from our laboratory instead of falling victim to the restrictions of our inner critic. Creative space is a consequence of truly practicing What's In the Way Is the Way. It acts as prolific mud for our lotus and it is how we get from buried to planted.

Back before I discovered yoga, when I was a singer/songwriter, I somehow managed to get invited to Joni Mitchell's fiftieth birthday party. It was in Venice Beach at just the sort of swanky artist's loft you would expect it to be—down an unassuming little side street and hidden behind an enormous concrete wall. Outdoor courtyard and spectacular indoor industrial square-footage with polished cement floors, giant bright colored artwork on the white walls, and one huge sectional couch were the only permanent design elements. Rented folding chairs littered the hip, minimalist landscape to accommodate partygoers who visited the outside bar and searched for a seat. Sound bounced off the extraordinarily high ceilings. Conversations comingled with Joni's "Got 'Til It's Gone" collaboration with Janet Jackson that played most of the evening. One of the first things Joni had us do when we arrived was take a dance lesson one group at a time. As if the evening weren't surreal enough, as I tried to learn to cha-cha, Harry Dean Stanton sat and watched me from his folding chair.

I'd spent an evening with Joni over dinner a few months before with mutual music friends. "You put down the skeleton, then you do the overdub. On a canvas, on a track, a bass line, or a sketch—it's all the same process," she explained. Her time in art school had inspired her to write music before lyrics. This was especially interesting from a lyrical icon. She said the more difficult puzzle of matching meter to melody made her most creative. Our talk motivated me to paint a birthday card for her, and when I presented it to her post cha-cha class she took me aside and said, "It's all the same, you know. Music, painting, poetry, it all comes from the same place. Do all of it."

*BOOM!*

I was encouraged, inspired, and more than a little overwhelmed. She represented an era and an integrity that seemed galaxies away from where my little artistic ventures could ever go. But she'd taken the time to tell me never to limit myself, and those words have not been forgotten.

There is composition in creating a yoga class too. It feels musical in moments, as if

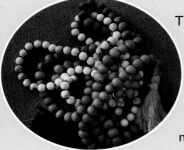

Tirumalai Krishnamacharya was a five-foot two-inch Brahmin born in 1888 in South India. His students include many of modern yoga's most notable teachers, such as his son T. K. V. Desikachar, Indra Devi (the only woman in the group), Sri K. Pattabhi Jois, and B. K. S. Iyengar. During the 1920s Krishnamacharya performed a lot of public demonstrations to generate attendance at his yoga school in Mysore, India. Among his exhibition favorites were: suspending his pulse, lifting heavy weights with his teeth, stopping cars barehanded, and performing impressive pretzel poses. These were the early years of the Indian independence movement, and Gandhi's ideals of ahimsa (non-violence) were a central part of India's struggle for freedom from the British Raj. Much of the Hindu, Sanskrit, and Indian traditions that had fallen away under the pressure of colonial rule were now finding their way back into Indian culture.

Krishnamacharya was considered a scholar of Indian medicine and disciplines such as Sanskrit, law, and ritual. His style of yoga asana (postures) was one that emphasized strength and stamina. Heavily influenced, no doubt, by the fact that most of his students at this point were active teenaged boys. Two of these teen boys were Pattabhi Jois and B. K. S. Iyengar. Jois is considered the father of Ashtanga yoga. Ashtanga is full of movement, whereas Iyengar's style of yoga moves much more slowly and emphasizes structural alignment—props like blocks, blankets, and belts are used to assist precise execution of the poses.

orchestrating a symphony in real time. I have to read the room and move with an intuitive current. Not unlike in my singing days, I stand in front of people and guide them with my voice. It's another example of what Joni was talking about—we let the creative juices flow through us in whatever form they appear. I draw from my mixed bag of yoga influences, my songwriting past, and my ongoing studies, but when I teach I feel like a conduit for something much larger than just little old me.

The movement of Ashtanga and the alignment of Iyengar are the primary foundations for what we have come to call vinyasa or flow yoga in the Western world. They are the classics, the straight-ahead jazz in a sea of neo-bop and acid jazz fusions. But in their very specific, traditional form, they may not speak to all of us who consider ourselves interested in yoga. Not everyone wants to listen to classical, or even classic rock all the time—some secretly yearn for a catchy pop song here and there. Not all of us are willing to play only by traditional rules, even if we respect their deep history. I'm not suggesting reckless impiety, only that we follow Joni's advice and let ourselves "do all of it." This freedom to explore allows us to form our own spiritual beliefs and find the type of postural yoga that speaks to us in a meaningful way. What resonates with one person may not with another (aggrotech music, anyone?).

For example, T. K. V. Desikachar believed that the practice needed to be individualized to the particular situation of each practitioner. He preferred one-on-one teaching to groups. I have private clients who share his opinion, and group class students who love it when it's mat-to-mat crowded and would rather fold their neighbor's laundry than practice alone with me. Some people love things like the kapalabhati (breath of fire) Kundalini offers, or chanting and kirtan, while others see that as reason to run swiftly in the other direction. There are many incredible styles and teachers to experiment with and experience out there.

Next to Joni, I felt almost like an artistic imposter. As I've developed my yoga teaching voice I've tangled with insecurities too. In an instant what feels like authentic creativity can career into the fear of being a pontificating poser. With a backdrop of five-thousand-year-old philosophy and modern-day postural offerings—weekend teacher training certificates to ninety-year-old master gurus—there are a lot of things out there claiming to be yoga. The question of what constitutes "real" yoga is a land mine I wander around carefully. Sometimes it can be very hard to see that it "all comes from the same place."

Tim Miller is one of the most gracious, humble people you'll meet. He was the first American certified to teach Ashtanga, and he runs the Ashtanga Yoga Center in Encinitas, California. Ashtanga is a rigorous sun salutation–drenched lineage of yoga said to have been derived from an ancient text called the *Yoga Korunta*. There are six different series in Ashtanga, and the student classically practices and progresses at his or her own pace, not in a led group class. The sequences are regimented, very specific, and performed in the same order for what is counted out as the same amount of breaths each time. Typically this practice takes place early in the morning, and lasts over two hours.

I don't happen to be an Ashtangi, but my teacher training with Tim (a year after my little local studio training) was a turning point for me. I was at first intimidated by the Ashtanga purist tribe who joined me in Tulum, Mexico, for our study. Initially I felt clumsy and reckless with my vinyasa vernacular and hodgepodge education, like an obnoxious dinner guest who keeps interrupting naturally flowing repartee with her mouth full. Or being surrounded by serious academics and realizing my liberal arts education was maybe a little *too* liberal (why, why so much time reading *Vogue* and so little Virgil?). But it was here as the self-proclaimed outcast, with the serious Ashtangis and Tim's generous guidance, that I learned to lighten up a bit and began to see how it all comes from the same place.

Gurus for thousands of years have been pointing to svadhyaya (self-study) as our fundamental learning tool. Svadhyaya is our individual collection of inspiring experiences, texts, teachings, and contemplations that act as a mirror for us to further understand ourselves. Whether it's inspiration from reading the Bible, Hindu texts, or the current *New York Times* best-selling self-help offering, the stillness of meditation or just turning off our phone, the guidance of a live teacher or an app, svadhyaya ultimately directs us toward a genuine sense of self. It isn't memorization; it's comprehension, and our individual recipe for self-reflection and growth.

I came to realize a couple of things in Tulum with Tim and the fundamentalists. First, when you trace it back, the postural yoga most of us are doing today comes from the same place. The second was that it didn't matter whether my yoga was in traditional packaging or unconventional garb, the materials we use come from the same place. After all, regardless of what we might prefer, "Oops! . . . I Did It Again" was built from the same harmonic scale as Joni's canonized "Both Sides Now." As teachers and as people we all ultimately come from the same place, though we're radically diverse in many ways. We can appreciate the choices and styles of others while we embrace our own.

In order to become abundantly creative in ways that allow us to reach our full potential, we need to be brave enough to *do all of it*. If you think about it, we're all in the process of composing the symphony, painting the picture, or writing the poem that is our life. Like Joni says, we want to encourage our inherent phrasings and visceral melodies from the broadest, most vibrant palette and vocabulary possible. Only then can we discover life's most fulfilling expression.

## ON YOUR MAT

No matter how inflexible your hips, shoulders, or hamstrings might be, I think where we're often the tightest is in our opinions. Just like our muscles enjoy a stretch, a bit of extension through our tightly wound ideas about things will open us up too. This **On Your Mat** is about moving your mat as well as moving on your mat. I've got a couple of "do all of it" yoga dates to help you reach out of the routine you might be a little bit too married to. I'm not a Hatha-home-wrecker. No one's asking you to abandon your loyalty to your chosen system, salutation, or sirsasana (headstand) forever. Just to create a little bit of creative space around what's already familiar. And as proof of my respect for observances, I want you to vow to spend time with your **Possibility Pose** regardless of where or with whom you might wake up from savasana this week.

1.  For the next week, I want you to agree to put your mat down in a new part of the room each time you practice. Whether that's for these postures we're doing here together, or when you head out to take class somewhere—I know, I know, you love your wall/corner/beloved back row, but changing the position of our mat also repositions us creatively—and you never know where that might lead. (I've had many students go from moving their mat in the room to unrolling it across the globe with me on retreat.)

2.  Take your mat on a blind date and step outside your usual yoga regimen for a moment. If you are a hard-core vinyasa practitioner, wander into an Iyengar class.

Never been to an Ashtanga, Restorative, Yin, Kundalini, Pranayama, or Hot Yoga class? Give one of those a go. Take a field trip to a class you've never taken before, dip your toe into a technique with which you are not yet acquainted. Be open-minded about your experiment. Worst-case scenario, you don't love it and are reminded of why you've landed on the style of yoga you do regularly. Even just going to a different studio to practice gives you a new vantage point.

Remember what Joni said—it all comes from the same place—but where it goes from there can be fascinating personal progress. Stepping outside of our norm and looking at things from a new angle feeds both our self-study (svadhyaya) and our creative space. It gives us a larger life canvas on which to paint our yoga.

## ON YOUR OM

You've felt Creating Space Is Creative Space from simply moving your mat—Becoming Bendy enough to try new styles and shift your perspective. In your yoga practice you've discovered Creative Space as length in your torso, allowing you to fold in a little deeper; in your breathing, giving you more comfort and ease; and in your meditation practice, developing further clarity and awareness. Now you'll see how your **Close to OM** evolution moves you toward open-minded perceptions that allow you to become receptive to the vivid colors Joni is talking about off your mat too.

Like your **On Your Mat** svadhyaya ingredients, your **On Your OM** self-study is your own recipe too. Val-you reminds us we aren't designing a formula to impress other people. We are courageously creating our own path. Creativity is often the result of diverse and even seemingly contrary elements. I mean, look at us. We are created from a combination of masculine and feminine—every breath we take opposing inhales and exhales. Hatha, an umbrella term used to describe the myriad practices of yoga asana and breathing, translates as "sun/moon" or balance of opposites. And our "do all of it" is an insightful paradox of intellectual and experiential—classical and current—concerned and hopeful. To be creative is to be brave enough to transcend the "what will people think" bullring of other people's opinions, labels, titles, and rules—to color outside the lines and design our own rodeo. We must muster the audacity to S.T.A.R.T. where we are right now. As the saying goes, "Courage is being scared to death but saddling up anyway."

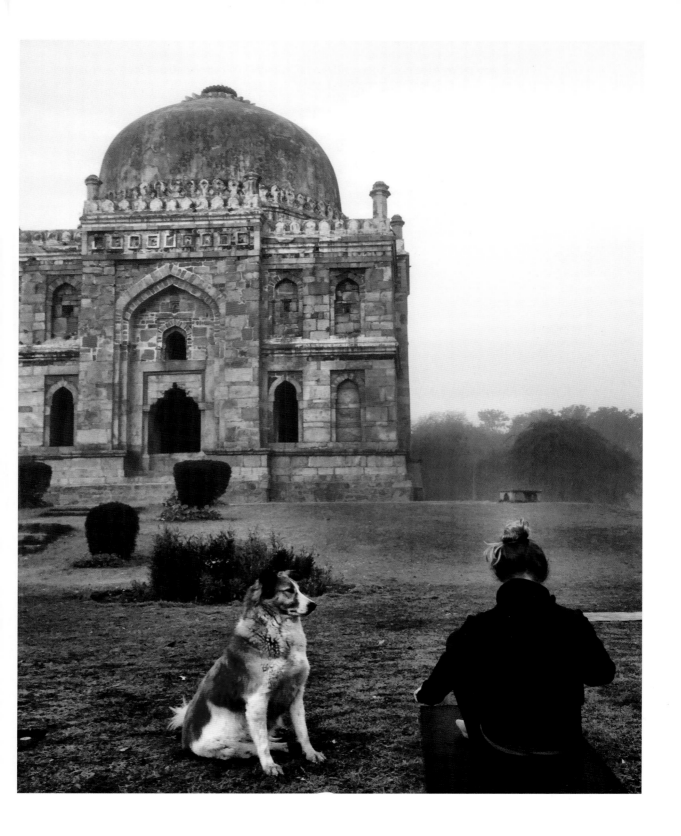

My mother, Gwen Marcum, owned the Book Café in Capitola, California, for thirty years. She worshiped the periodicals and had zero patience for the self-help section. Why anyone would feel the need to talk about feelings was beyond her. Joseph "Follow Your Bliss" Campbell, Wayne "The Power of Intention" Dyer, Louise "You Can Heal Your Life" Hay were the stuff of her nightmares. There were a few other random things she had strong opinions about, for example, vacations. What would possess a person to go somewhere to relax and do nothing when they could be home accomplishing things like ironing shirts and preparing dinner? She did, however, see value in travel, as long as we stayed somewhere long enough to learn something.

My junior year in high school, Gwen set her sights on France. While our father stayed home in Santa Cruz and worked, Mama, my brothers Eddy and Art, and I created a do-it-yourself semester abroad program. One she felt no need to clear with any of our American schools.

First stop: Paris.

To say that Gwen's French was limited would be kind. It wasn't just that she had no vocabulary or syntax, her accent was so far off no one could understand the few things she could say. That by some miracle she was able to find her friend Phyllis's apartment in the ninth arrondissement turned her three children into "The Power Of Intention" believers, even if she wasn't. We spent much of our first days in Paris at the French Open tennis tournament so that we would "stay out of Phyllis's hair." In fact, my mom used the Open as a bit of a babysitter, leaving my too-young-to-be-left-alone brothers for stretches of hours while she wandered with me out into the city. Butchering French at every turn, we frantically compiled semester-at-sea options. She decided we would head to the Mediterranean resort town of Cap d'Agde.

Now hold on. Just in case you're encouraged that we might finally be heading to the vacation we never had, let me just say one thing: off-season. It was fall when we arrived, and a ghost town. All that was left of the good times of summer were vomit stains and the occasional abandoned flip-flop.

Somehow, Gwen had managed to locate Club de Tennis Pierre Barthes where Eddy could continue his tennis training. There was also an elementary school for Art. Other than that there wasn't much going on in off-season Cap d'Agde. We listened to our two cassette tapes: AC/DC *Back in Black* and the London recording of *Evita*, over and over again. And to our only neighbors fighting in heavy Cockney accents about sausages and beans. I tried to attend the local high school, but with my French only slightly better than Gwen's it was not quite the right fit.

So Gwen figured out how I could be an au pair in Paris for an American actress with two little boys from a French director ex-husband, and her new French movie actor boyfriend who lived downstairs. The assignment was less about a grueling nanny schedule, and more about being responsible for myself for the first time. I went to school at the Alliance Française and took claquettes (tap dancing) and jazz dance classes at the American Center. I turned sixteen and yearned for my driver's license back home, but knew that what I was doing was probably more expansive. In retrospect I see it as one of the most formative times of my life and a model for my future svadhyaya.

Gwen Marcum is terrified of freeway driving, airplane travel, and not sounding smart enough at dinner parties. She's incapable of accepting a compliment. But underneath it all, she's one of the bravest, most exceptional people I know. I'm not sure I'd have the guts to take my kids out of the country the way she did. She fought fiercely throughout our childhoods to find adventurous and often unorthodox opportunities for us.

On the door of our bathroom in Santa Cruz, Mama taped the words "HUSTLE MAKES IT HAPPEN." It was her mantra. Yes, words like *bliss* and *joyful* made her stomach turn, but *hustle* was the gospel. Some like their "do all of it" sanguine and celestial, while others need a bit more grit and heavy lifting. In the end, the semantics and delivery don't matter as much as the actual doing. Whether it's hustle or self-help—personal best or finding your true north—it's about making it happen. Gwen Marcum made it happen.

I'm not saying you have to immediately quit your job, pull your kids out of school, put everything in storage, and travel abroad to add new colors to your gray. But I am saying you don't have to wait until you have millions of dollars, the perfect plan, perfect body, an impressive degree, or your hairdresser's approval to be creative. You just have to remain curious. Remember, "You don't have to throw a single punch to be boxing" . . . but you need to do the footwork. Maybe today's versa-climber class leads you to the top of Machu Picchu some day, that stationary spin bike becomes the S.T.A.R.T. of an eighty-mile life-changing AIDS ride, or the book on tape you've been listening to during your walk leads you to a new career. I've seen it happen more than a few times. I mean, what if that yoga class you almost didn't take at your gym twenty years ago ends up inspiring a book published by St. Martin's Press one day?

Take a different route to work, order something new for lunch, listen to a different radio station, or peruse the local paper for events and happenings to go to.

Pull out your notebook and look at the exercise you did when you took accountability for your **Stuckat List** and answered:

1.  How did my actions contribute to this situation?

You are now going to apply Joni's "do all of it" creativity to the following question:

2.  How can I contribute to a solution?

For example, say you had "**Stuckat** wasting my day in the car sitting in traffic" on your list. Take your beginner's mind for a spin. Download something interesting so that you can plug it in and listen while en route. Make your drive time inspired time. Learn a new language. Listen to somebody's biography. Immerse yourself in interviews and lectures on topics you've meant to investigate. Become Bendy behind the wheel and feel innovation steering you **Close to OM**.

Maybe you feel stuck in a relationship that isn't working anymore . . . with a person? Yourself? Food? Your job? A substance? Exercise? Can you S.T.O.P. and S.T.A.R.T. to see What's In the Way Is the Way to create a new relationship? Can Val-you help you out of the bullring of self-loathing and into a rodeo full of nourishing potentials? In my workshops, people have reframed being buried under the job they hate and turned it into a way to be planted. They've realized the income from where they're working now can be the financial seeds for what they are growing next: going into business for themselves, paying for photography school, studying to be a product manager, funding that expensive yoga teacher training . . . Your current job is only the enemy if you make it that way. Your interpretation can turn what feels like **Stuckat** into a creative "do all of it" launching pad.

Like the little savasanas and ABCs you're taking throughout the day, what small manageable steps can you take toward a **Stuckat** solution? It's important to be playful as you come up with ideas. Having fun doesn't mean that you're not being productive.

Maybe there are things you used to love to do that for some reason you've stopped. Begin again, pay close attention, and reintroduce yourself to the joys of tasting, feeling, hearing, smelling, and seeing those things that made you feel alive. Take off your shoes and feel the sand between your toes, rub a few drops of that essential oil you love between your palms and sit for a moment to enjoy the aroma, make a date with yourself to go see that exhibit you were curious about, join a book club, a knitting circle, a run club, a gardening class, do the crossword puzzle, learn to write haiku. Get back into the routine of filling up your fridge with delightful farmer's market produce that feeds a healthy, happy relationship with food instead of **Stuckat** the drive-thru. Bring some of your farmer's market loot, or a plant from your gardening class, to the neighbor you've been fighting with to S.T.A.R.T. the process of improving that relationship too. **Stuckat** solutions can be serious fun, but just like your **Possibility Pose** and breathing meditations, you have to actually follow through in order to create space for them in your life. You have to actually do it.

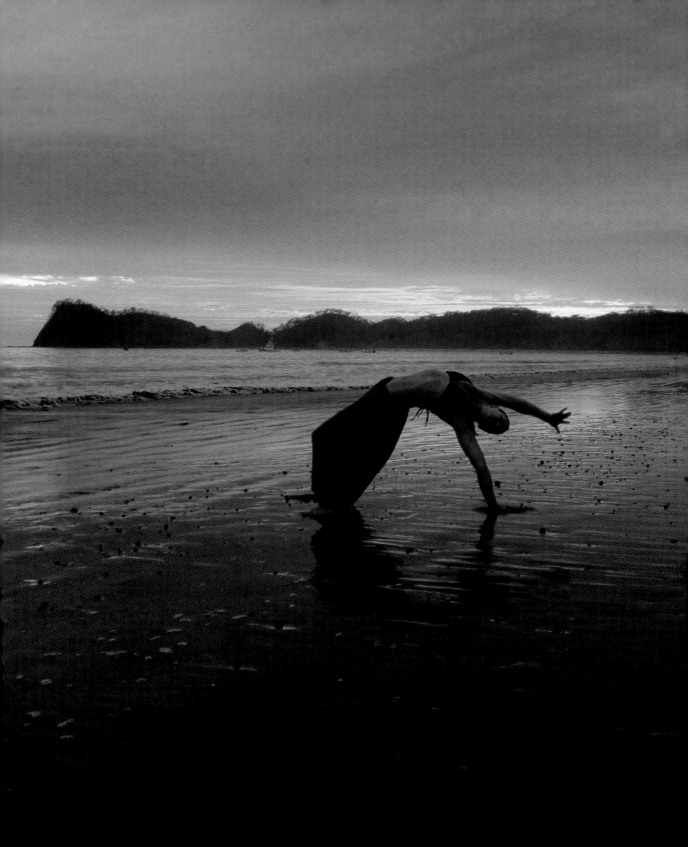

# PART III

# UNITE

You might say the emphasis in *awaken* and *transform* is mind and body, whereas on this leg of your journey you *unite* with spirit. You look at compassion, intuition, and integrity and create connections to your highest, greatest self. It is here that you fully realize "how you do your yoga is how you do your life." It is where you find your **OM**.

# 12

# Compassion

*Love and compassion are necessities,*

*not luxuries. Without them humanity*

*cannot survive.*

—DALAI LAMA

**In this chapter you *unite* with compassion. You discover ahimsa as part of your path toward peace and acceptance within your Self and those around you.**

It can be very easy to judge.

We think we've got everybody all figured out, but the labels we point to in order to explain who we are often have little to do with core qualities.

Take, for example, compassion.

Vegetarians, Environmentalists, Yogis, Parents: all of these labels suggest people who naturally exhibit a lot of compassion, right? What then of non-yoga-practicing, carnivorous, climate change–denying real estate developers—are they completely devoid of compassion? Nothing is black or white in this life, especially when we are talking about our inner life. It is slippery terrain when we start equating types of people with specific qualities. As a result, we all might have a little trouble seeing the hypocrite in the mirror if we aren't careful.

For the longest time I was insecure about the fact that I didn't have kids. I sensed sideways looks from society at large, and a need to explain myself. I felt like I was wearing a giant sign that read "LACKS COMPASSION FOR ANYONE BUT MYSELF."

So I would try too hard.

I held the babies and read books to the kids who wanted nothing to do with me to make up for my lack of procreation. Desperate to appear kid-friendly, I would buy too many presents for everyone else's kids, donate immediately to their school fundraiser, and buy ridiculous amounts of Girl Scout cookies and overpriced candy drive chocolate bars. Proof that I was near kids, even if I was not producing them. The exhausted parents would watch me from the sidelines, and I was convinced they were annoyed by my free time to do the things I wanted, clean car, and stories of international travel. I sensed behind their glares, however, the smug conviction that they had the upper hand. They were the social norm, and they knew a love I never would.

But wait a minute.

Are the non-yoga-practicing, carnivorous, climate change–denying real estate developers and I really condemned to the No Compassion Corner?

What is it that defines compassion?

From its Latin stem, compassion is defined as "the ability for a person to feel what the other person is feeling." If you look it up in a modern dictionary, it's mostly associated with grief and sympathy. But its origins suggest "feeling with each other" in ways that are more expansive than just feeling sorry for each other. Compassion is our way to see things from another's perspective. Having kids certainly affords us that opportunity. So do our chosen spiritual and religious paths. Problems occur when we harden around the ego aspects of our choices and become righteous and judgmental. Our religion is right and yours is wrong. Our lifestyle is right and yours is wrong. We suffocate compassion with our ego's need to be right. If you tease this behavior out onto the global stage, you have far more damaging consequences. These angry embers become the flames that cause conflict and even killing. It can be shocking to see how seemingly innocuous the seed was that inspired the eventual horror.

It is through compassion that we find peace. The Bible, the Koran, the Bhagavad Gita, and other religious texts all ultimately espouse compassion. However, our personal insecurities and inadequacies (our lack of Val-you) can fuel our prejudices, making it difficult to let compassion unfold in our lives. It's very hard to arrive at compassion for others if we cannot arrive at it in ourselves. This sounds a lot fluffier than it actually is. I know it from my own experience, but I see it in the classroom all the time. The mat is a microcosm for more universal behavior. We get frustrated that someone a few mats down is doing something that we can't. Defeated by our limitations and somehow threatened by their abilities, our ego bursts. With our self-esteem boat sinking, we look desperately for chinks in their armor. Putting them down gives us a false sense of elevating ourselves. But like forcing an injured shoulder too far into a stretch, our aggressive and hurtful attitude only creates more suffering and pain. We make ourselves crazy trying to direct everyone and everything toward something we hope makes us seem better than they are. And, just like that we've forgotten to lose the competition.

Compassion keeps us on course and moves us **Close to OM**.

*Ahimsa* is a word both Hindus and Buddhists use as the basis for compassion. Patanjali cites it in his *Yoga Sutras* as part of a path to a more peaceful existence. It connotes unconditional acceptance and friendship with oneself and an active interest in others.

"Compassion makes us dethrone ourselves from the center of our world, and put another there," says esteemed author and theologian Karen Armstrong. Not only is that something we can all practice, it is something that we must do for the survival of our global dysfunctional family. We have to find our way to a place where we feel less threatened and more thoughtful. We don't have to agree, but we must accept that there are a lot of different ways of doing things and that they can coexist.

Warren Buffett loves his philanthropy along with his steak and his Cherry Coke. Ron Terwilliger, head of Trammell Crow Residential, one of the largest developers of multifamily housing in the U.S., is also the recipient of the Hearthstone Builder Humanitarian Award and has donated $100 million to Habitat for Humanity. There are plenty of parents in the world who cannot seem to muster compassion for someone else's child, sometimes even their own. And some of our icons for compassion like Mother Theresa and the Dalai Lama had no children of their own.

The bottom line is, it's not our title, appearance, or wealth that defines whether we are compassionate or not, it is our actions. I often tell people that I do, in fact, have kids—some of them in their 60s and 70s. Working with the wonderful students I am blessed with dethrones me on a daily basis. As Rebecca Solnit says in her *Harper's Magazine* article entitled "The Mother of All Questions," "There are so many things to love besides one's own offspring, so many things that need love, so much other work love has to do in the world."

Judith Hanson Lasater is one of yoga's pioneering women. She asked me when I interviewed her, "Why are we doing all these handstands, backbends, and arm balances?" She doesn't understand why we're doing them unless they shape and change our lives. "I believe that yoga should lead us to a place where kindness and compassion are instantaneous. Compassion is fierce and strong, and it holds people accountable. But it doesn't do it with anger or judgment. I don't think we find compassion. I think we become the space that compassion wants to live in. You can't make yourself *be* compassionate, you can only keep stepping back and becoming a larger container in which compassion wants to live."

In other words, Creating Space Is Creative *and* Compassionate Space.

## ON YOUR MAT

Taking creative action is liberating but can feel vulnerable too. That's why compassion is key. It's easy to limit yoga asana (poses) to just the body aspect of body/mind/spirit, but as you've seen in these pages, asana leads us to a more conscious and less reactive way of living too. Asana is a powerful gateway to ahimsa (compassion). What better time to remind ourselves of generosity than when we feel wobbly, impatient, weak, or tight—least likely to exhibit grace and awareness in a pose? In our postures as in life, it's easy to be considerate when everything is going well, but it becomes magnanimous when it

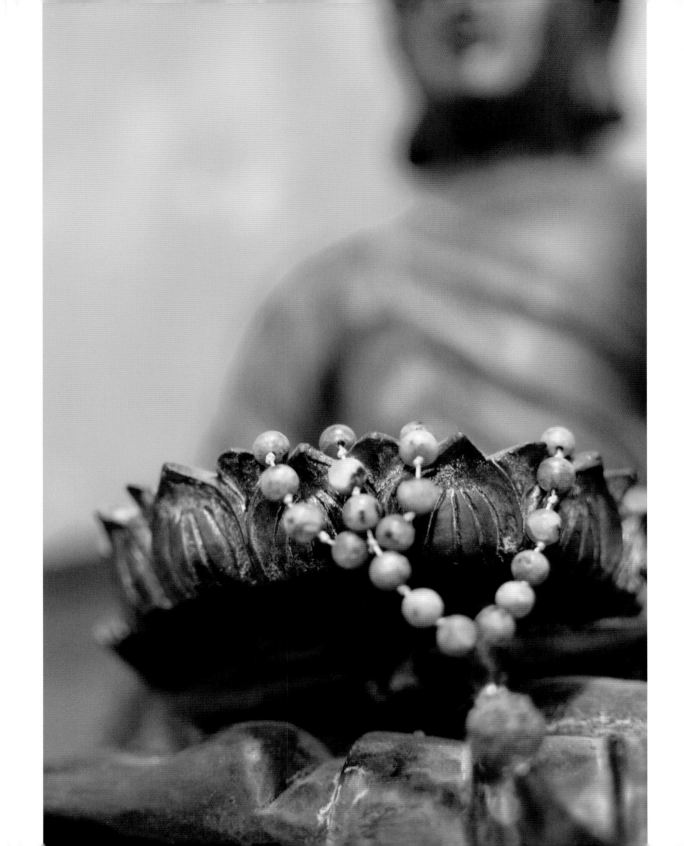

blossoms amid the rubble. Compassion for our own foibles lends itself to a similar compassion toward others.

Earlier you were invited to make some changes—to Become Bendy enough to move your mat location in the room, choose alternate versions of your poses, and even to visit different studios and classes. Now I ask that you see those inspirations as more than fleeting isolated events. Allow them to be the impetus for real transformation. Just as we have to want to learn, we have to be willing to be creatively and compassionately consistent. As our **Possibility Pose** has been proving, most change is incremental and occurs over a committed stretch of time. We want to *unite* change with transformation to allow it to make us wiser, kinder, and stronger.

The immediacy of a posture reminds us to S.T.A.R.T. right here right now with creativity, compassion, consistency, and commitment (you might remember them as the Four Cs). The physiology of our asana is the most tangible layer (kosha) of our Self to access. Somatic (bodily) sensations are straightforward messengers that *unite* us instantly with the opportunity to see what's really going on. I think balancing poses are particularly fantastic laboratories for our Four Cs. Let's use vrikshasana (tree pose) as an example. Compassion acts as deep roots for our tree . . . you'll see.

Our tree grows out of our mountain (tadasana). With both feet evenly standing on your mat (samasthiti), place your hands on your chest to find your even breathing (sama vritti). S.T.O.P. to S.T.A.R.T. and appreciate the ABCs of your breathing—feel free to add the ujjayi textured sound to your breath here too.

Shift all your weight into your left foot and bring the bottom of your right foot into the inseam of your left thigh, calf, or even ankle. Flexibility will have something to do with where this right foot ends up for you. It's important not to feel that one expression of the pose is better than the other. We're all unique combinations of genes, strength, balance, and pliability. You yourself will be different depending on the day, what you've eaten, any injuries you're working through, how much sleep you did or didn't get, et cetera. Over time and through the seasons, our trees will assume variegated shapes and forms. Enjoy your laboratory. Get excited about wearing your own genes, not frustrated by trying to fit into someone else's.

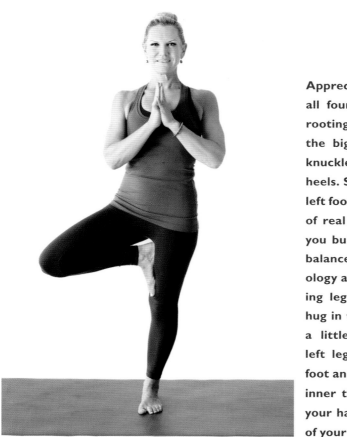

Appreciate the experience of all four points of your left foot rooting your tree into the soil—the big toe knuckle, pinkie toe knuckle, and inner and outer heels. Since this small but mighty left foot of yours is not a whole lot of real estate to stand on, what you build above it is essential to balance—both in terms of physiology and focus. Tone your standing leg by feeling the outer hip hug in toward the midline. Sense a little energetic dance—outer left leg toward bottom of right foot and bottom of right foot into inner thigh, calf, or ankle. Bring your hands into a prayer in front of your heart.

Find ekagrata—single pointed focus—gazing at one point either right out at the horizon or, if it's helpful for balance, down toward the ground. Our drishti (concentration point) is our way of looking out while turning our awareness inward, our way of seeing the forest for the trees. Stay as long as you can on this first side, and then try the same configuration on side two.

We're going to embark upon some playful compassion, creativity, consistency, and commitment using vrikshasana as our guide. With each of these creative add-ons, find a healthy dose of compassion as gusts of wind inevitably challenge your commitment and most likely huff and puff and blow your tree down from time to time. (You'll find this as audio instruction @OM too.)

From our basic formation above:

1.  Try extending the branches of your tree to the sky.

2.  Shift your gaze up to your extended branches.

3.  Play with coming on to the tippy toes of your standing foot as if you were wearing very impractical high heels—combine that with your gaze to the sky.

4.  Still standing? Try closing your eyes . . .

Know that consistency will bring connections and a better understanding of your balance, body, brain, and botanical bravura. Plant your tree next to your **Possibility Pose** for the next two weeks and watch it grow. If we use our yoga for more than just a workout, it will educate us far beyond our muscles and bones. It will guide us toward ahimsa (compassion), aparigraha (non-greediness), and asteya (enough Val-you and faith to believe we can create our own instead of stealing from others). We may never be able to balance on our tippy toes with our eyes closed, but we just might be able, one day in the Four C-able (as a reminder, The Four Cs are creativity, compassion, consistency, and commitment) future to thank our challenges and adversaries for what we've learned about compassion.

Be sure to luxuriate in a five-minute savasana once you're done climbing in your tree—a constitutional reminder that deep roots support our widening branches.

## ON YOUR OM

When you start to take a more expansive look at your life, it's easiest to determine what you don't want. "I don't want to be waiting tables anymore when I'm thirty. I don't want to keep dating assholes. I don't want to be a burden. I don't want to sound like my mother. I don't want to end up like so-and-so." In other words, much of what you find on your **Stuckat List**. But you don't want to stay stuck at **Stuckat**.

You've made a list of what you *don't* want, and now you're going to wander in even deeper and write down what you *do* want. This is big. This is you crossing over from your **Stuckat List** to what you might call your **OM Stretch**. In posture-speak this is that moment when you have the bravery to commit to doing your headstand in the middle of the room instead of using the excuse that you "didn't use the wall," even though you're still parked in front of it.

Now to be clear, this is not a list of what you want to steal from others. It's what you want to create that's authentically your own. And it's not made of spite, lies, jealousy, hatred, revenge, or backbiting. The introduction of compassionate philosophy to my yoga practice led me to a spot in the fence where I could peek through and see there was another way. Three concepts I mentioned earlier changed my course from the bullring of envy, blame, greed, and punishment—major ways in which I was stuck—to a rodeo full of compassion.

Ahimsa literally translates as non-violence. It also suggests that punishing ourselves with desires so far-fetched that they queue us up for feeling inadequate, inept, and less-than is a form of violence too. For example, if what we want is to be ten years younger, six inches taller, a PhD, and an Olympic gold medalist by the next week, and all rainy days to be sunny, we are failing to embrace the thoughtful precepts of ahimsa.

Asteya (non-stealing) is our ability to find fulfillment within that which comes to us by honest means. What is ours will find us in its own extraordinary way if we make room for it.

Aparigraha (non-greediness) means not clinging to anything that rings untrue. Conforming to traditions or expectations that are not our own prevent us from what Patanjali's *Yoga Sutras* calls a "life without undue burden, free to be who you are." It also means non-greediness in a more material or external way, not hoarding things that are not needed. Aparigraha reminds us that achieving elaborate poses or the trappings of conventional success will not necessarily bring us happiness and contentment.

Before introducing yoga into my life, I was under the false impression that other people were getting what I deserved—that their triumphs were coming out of my pocket. But as I did the work you are doing now, I began to see that if someone else met a man, fell in love, and got married, she wasn't taking my guy, she had merely found hers. And women with obnoxiously long, thick, beautiful, "good" hair hadn't stolen what I was supposed to get, either.

Take a moment to become present before putting pen to paper (or fingers on the keys). S.T.O.P. to S.T.A.R.T.—then *unite* with creative space and courageous compassion as you honestly record your vision for what you really want. You will be adding to this over time as things occur to you. Like you did with your tree. You establish your trunk so that you can explore new branches.

# 13

# From Your Head to Your Heart

*Blessed are the hearts that can bend;*

*they shall never be broken.*

—ALBERT CAMUS

**In this chapter you learn that to *unite* with OM means trading intellect for intuition sometimes. It means shifting from your head to your heart.**

As I mentioned, courageous creativity leaves us feeling a bit exposed, which is amplified as we move past our **Stuckat List** and really own the life we want. Creativity is like love. It's a leap of faith that asks us to be daring and step into the unknown. Sometimes that calls for less intellect and more intuition.

When I first opened U Studio, I was the only teacher. That meant seven days a week with no time off in sight. But when you're getting started, you're just grateful people are actually crossing your threshold. A few months in, I finally got up the nerve to sub out my very first class to attend a wedding. A couple of students who'd come to my class on their first date invited me, and though I was terrified to leave my studio kids with a sitter (and almost didn't) I went.

I didn't know Renee and Doug very well, and therefore didn't really know anyone at their wedding either. But Renee's Canadian family was warm and easygoing and loved their ABBA on the dance floor. They were the antithesis of LA's tendency toward phony and pretentious. I fell for them instantly. We danced the night away under the stars at a country club I'd never known existed on Sepulveda near the Getty Museum.

At the coffee wagon, getting espresso and biscotti for his nonna, I met Renee's brother Dom. He was a man's man, in a classy gray suit with a neatly cropped goatee and wonderful deep voice. We talked and talked, and joined the rest of the family for a second round of "Dancing Queen" and "Fernando." At one point he put his hand on the small of my back.

"Never take that away," I thought to myself. It just felt like it belonged there.

"Don't be silly," was my next thought. He lived thousands of miles away and was only in town for a couple of days. It made no practical sense, and I had a new business to learn how to run. When he asked if I would go out to a bar with him after the wedding, I declined—I had an eight o'clock class the next morning and it was past midnight.

A baseball-loving, linebacker-sized ironworker from just over the Detroit boarder, Dominic Robert Pietrangelo was not exactly a yoga enthusiast. So when he showed up to take my class the following morning, I knew it wasn't his love of vinyasa that brought him there. I was floored that he would make such a brave gesture to see me again. Mine is known as one of the more challenging yoga classes in town, and he had no idea what he was in for. Evidently in *his* first down dog, he muttered to himself, "I need a beer" . . . a true Canadian.

After class, I could tell he needed a little encouragement. "Here's my number if you guys end up doing anything later," I volunteered so he wouldn't have to ask.

When I left my 4:00 p.m. class I found four voice mails awaiting me. Like the scene in the movie *Swingers*, Dom started by explaining that they were making dinner reservations, and I was welcome to join them, but I didn't have to. The next added the time of the reservations to "you don't have to" . . . then the suggested attire . . . where I could park. It was like he had found himself caught in voice mail quicksand and couldn't find anything to hold on to that would make it stop.

The Magic Castle has been a Hollywood institution since 1963. It's a bit like a musty haunted-house amusement park ride with very serious magicians and expensive steak dinners. As I drove up their driveway, there was Dom at the valet station in his dress-code-required dinner jacket (the one he'd been wearing the night before) waiting for me. I'd assumed the newly married couple we knew in common were the "we" in the dinner reservation, but I was wrong. Instead his great aunt Angela, his cousin Lucy, and her husband Enzo were our Italian chaperones.

The quicksand Dom had combated earlier in the day had turned to verbal cement. He sat silently through dinner as the Italians and I finished each other's sentences like long lost migliore amicos. After dinner we all made our way into the Palace of Mystery and the hand that had rested on the small of my back at the wedding reached over to hold mine. The magic around us couldn't compare. It was ridiculously sweet, innocent, and fantastic. Don't get me wrong. We left the Magic Castle, said good night to the Italians, and proceeded to make out like teenagers in my car until it was time for Dom's flight.

The next day, when I recounted the events of the evening to my pal Tamara, she pulled her car over, got a catch in her throat, and said, "Oh my God, you're going to marry this guy." Now, not only does that sound like dialogue from a Lifetime cable movie, it was also obviously way too early in the story for marriage. But Tamara has always been a bit clairvoyant. She heard something new in my voice that she'd never heard before. Not in all of our years of friendship.

Yoga and the work you and I are doing together in this book had helped me get out of my head and land in my heart. Not the heart you find in an anatomy book—a more expansive heart, a compassionate space for love, creativity, and insight. Had I insisted on what "made sense" I would not be Mrs. Pietrangelo today. I was beginning to recognize my Val-you. I'd become someone who was attracting something different. Finally I'd manifested a man willing to chase me down and take me to dinner instead of someone who'd never even bothered to take me to coffee but was somehow living with me rent-free. I was no longer looking for someone to save me. I was ready for someone who deserved me.

## ON YOUR MAT

Have you ever noticed your posture when you're stuck in your head? Shoulders slumped forward and probably creeping up in your ears. Spine rounded, often arms crossed in front of your caved-in chest. It's as if your head has convinced you to bury your heart too deep to be found. Asana takes us from closed-off to consciously connected—body, mind, and spirit.

We're going to perform a little open-heart sequencing.

It would be ideal for you to start with five sun salutation As as a warm-up before we dive in. This is an especially good idea if it's cold or early in the morning. Refer back to page 42 or look at appendix 1 for a refresher and know that you'll find audio surya namaskar As @OM.

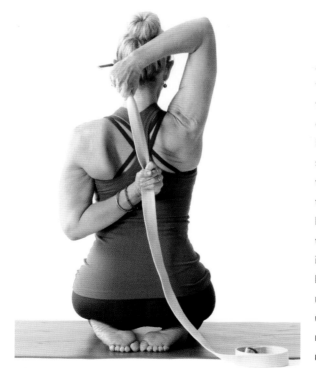

**After your As you're going to find virasana (page 104). This is a perfect time to revisit viveka (staying out of the bullring) as you fashion your seat. We're going to add some arm movements to this posture, so I highly recommend sitting on something—a block, folded blanket/towel, or pillow; even if that's on your heels (vajrasana)—instead of trying to force your sit bones to the ground. Remember, read this breakdown first, then use @OM as your audio guide or make your way back through the material on your own.**

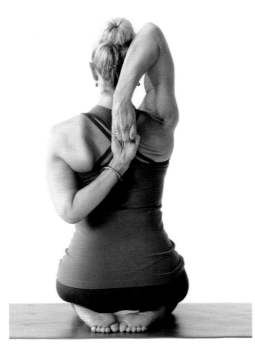

We'll start by adding gomukhasana arms to your virasana/vajrasana seat. Take your right arm straight up to the sky. Then imagine you have an itch in between your shoulder blades that you want to scratch with your right hand, inching that hand down your back with your elbow pointing skyward. Reach your left arm straight out to the side like half of a letter T. Bend at the elbow, fingers facing down. Start to move your bent left arm toward your body as if reaching your left hand up your spine to shake hands with your right.

Most of us will benefit from using a strap or a towel here to maneuver into tight shoulders. As much as your body will allow, migrate your elbows toward each other, hugging the midline of your spine. Notice if your top elbow is crushing your chin toward your chest and back off a little if it is. Think of making this elegant, spacious, and easeful, even if you feel a bit like you're in bondage. Stay here for at least six cycles of breath. Then release and find the second side of your gomukhasana arms. Feel free to shift a block under your seat or give your legs a break between sides if you need it. You're going to stay in this leg position a bit longer.

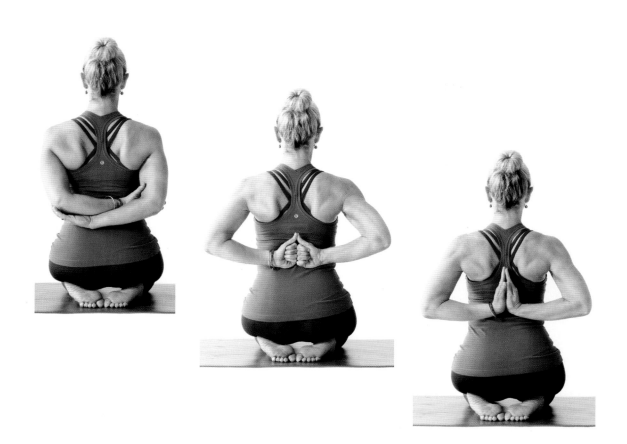

Remaining in vajrasana or virasana (seated on or between your feet), take both arms out to the side like a letter **T**. Bend both elbows, fingers facing down (think scarecrow position) and with your palms facing behind you, start to bring your two hands together behind your back. This is going to look and feel different on each of us. For some of you clasping elbows is the answer.

The other option is pressing fists together behind your back. Eventually, you'll make a prayer behind your back, pressing your palms together. Don't get overly concerned about what your hands are able to do today. Be more interested in what's happening in your shoulders and neck and how wide open your collarbones are becoming. Feel your prayer, or semblance of a prayer, lifting your heart and allow your shoulders to open as you find tadasana (mountain pose) in your torso and the calm of a savasana . . . even if your prayer is for this to be over soon.

After six full cycles of breath, carefully release your arms, slide out of your virasana seat, and come onto your belly. Make a pillow out of your hands and rest your head to one side. Take note of your wide, deep breathing against the ground here. Try to narrow your breath down to through the nose and not the mouth, and consider folding in the sound and texture of ujjayi if you haven't already.

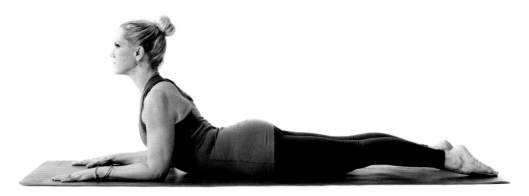

**From here, lift up onto your forearms.**

Think back to our cobra at the beginning of the book and how it was all about length. With the awareness of our core work, draw your navel toward your spine, finding a light corseting action at the waist that will provide support for your extension. Press down into the tops of your feet and elongate your legs so much that your kneecaps come off your mat (but your feet stay down). As if you could make them move, pull your elbows back toward your chest, and let that action lift your heart forward through the gateway of your arms—almost like you're trying to drag yourself off the front end of your mat. Enjoy the imprint of your shoulder blades and let them contribute to the ascent of your heart. Stay here in sphinx pose for six cycles of breath, then release. You're welcome to take another round or two. Then make that pillow with your hands and rest your head to the opposite side from last time. Check in once again with your breath.

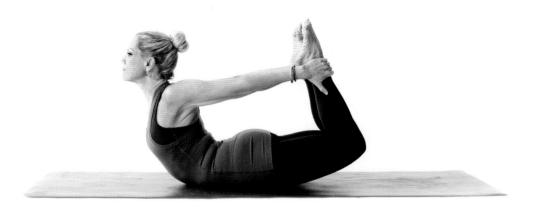

**Still lying on your stomach, bend your knees and reach back for your feet or ankles. If actually taking hold is not in the stars today, not to worry. Just bend your knees and pretend to hold on, or maybe lasso your feet or shins with a strap or towel.**

Find the lift of your navel for support, remember that feeling of lengthening your heart in sphinx, add the extension of your legs even as you hold onto your feet, and grow a very long bow pose (dhanurasana). Your legs are the power source here as they kick up and back, and will determine the level of intensity. Stay three to six full cycles of breath and carefully release. If you'd like to give it a few more rounds, great! We'll meet back in child's pose once you're done.

From child's pose you're going to come kneeling. Be sure to use padding under your knees if they're tender. A blanket or towel should do the trick, and curling your toes under might be helpful too. Remember how delicate and complicated your knees are. Don't piss them off: they always have the last word if you do. Find tadasana as you stand on your knees here. Imagine that you have a block in the inseams of your thighs and that you're trying to spit that block out behind you, creating what's called a neutral rotation. (By the way, you're welcome to actually use a block here if you have one.) Place your thumbs on your sacrum (the boney triangle at the base of your spine) with your fingers fanning out a bit.

Lift your navel to your spine like you did when you were on your belly, and think of gently brushing your hip bones against an invisible wall in front of you. Then, as if going up and over a barrel, extend backward into camel pose (ustrasana). No need to throw your head back or force yourself into the depths. Remember the bow pose you just did on your belly moments ago and ease toward a similar understanding of creating length in your spine—certain not to pinch or force anything in your low back or neck. Be sure you're breathing the whole time. If I were in the room with you, the magnitude of the pose should not be too much for you to muster a response if I asked you where you got your cool yoga pants. Stay for a few cycles of breath and with your belly firm come upright, then sit on your heels in vajrasana or between your heels in virasana if it's really comfortable for you.

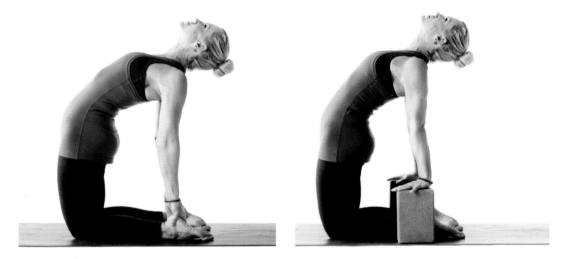

**At some point you might reach back with both hands for your heels in this pose.**

**That tends to be a lot easier to do with your toes curled under. It's not something to struggle to accomplish, just a variation to play with, perhaps. Another great trick is to use blocks on either side of your ankles.**

There are all sorts of nutty versions of this posture, including one where you place your head on the ground and grab your feet (kapotasana). But for our purposes today, ustrasana and the rest of our backbends are simply intended to lead us away from closed-off and overthinking, toward our center of creative energy and intuitive vs. intellectual perception. They act as an immediate, physical experience of how we limit ourselves with our static, fixed posturing. And they are an intrinsic reveal that there is another way, if we are willing, that will open us up to the whole of our heart.

When you're done playing with your ustrasana variations, take a pause in child's pose to regroup.

Then give yourself a few moments for a heartfelt tree and **Possibility Pose** visit.

Be sure to finish with the deliciousness of a five-minute savasana.

(You can find this full sequence as the Head To the Heart practice @**OM** and in appendix 1.)

## ON YOUR OM

To truly invite courageous creativity into our hearts and not just into our minds we have to be willing to move from stoic and academic to imaginative and visceral. Away from the kind of overthinking that would have had me **Stuckat** logic vs. love in my Dom story. Stepping boldly into what we want requires adventuring into our hearts and going on a bit of an intuitive rendezvous. You might say we need to vibrate at a higher frequency. (Settle down, I'm from Santa Cruz, I'm allowed to say things like "vibrate at a higher frequency" from time to time.)

This isn't limited to romantic love by the way. Let's say stepping into what you want has more of a corporate ring to it for you. The root of *corporate* is the Latin word *corpus*, which means body. To truly embody your Val-you on the job is to incorporate (there's that root word again) *awaken, transform,* and *unite* into your mission statement. Bernie Marcus and Arthur Blank had just been fired from their jobs when they followed their hearts instead of the myriad doubts in their heads to build Home Depot from scratch. Blake Mycoskie followed his belief to *Start Something That Matters* (the title of his book) when he created TOMS. Mel and Patricia Ziegler turned their crazy passion for safari wear into Banana Republic. By definition, a corporation is a group of people acting as one body—a body that requires visionary guts and a daring heart to act as the creative pulse and esprit de corps of innovation.

Committing to these next few exercises might at first seem awkward. They are going to take you on a less linear adventure and ask you to be resourceful in ways that may at first strike you as goofy. I was pretty snarky around them initially too. But I find myself leaning into them time and time again to stay **Close to OM** and I now enjoy them as much as I rely upon them. They also happen to be terrific building blocks for what we will dig into further in our next chapter.

1. Write yourself a letter as the person who has made their list of wants a reality. Be detailed about how it feels, looks, sounds, smells, tastes, etc. You can even put a stamp on it and mail it to yourself. Open it up and read it when you feel you need a friendly reminder. It's important that you actually do this one, as we will be returning to it later in the book.

2. Make a vision board. Collect pictures, words, phrases (you name it) that are visual reminders of what you want.

3. Create a playlist of songs that keep you inspired, focused on what you want, and totally invested in "where we put our focus is where we put our energy and where we put our energy is what manifests."

4. Record your list of wants. Listen to what it is that you want to invite into your life as you are preparing for your day, cleaning house, walking on the treadmill, driving, before you go to sleep—whenever. This not only acts as a reminder, it's also a powerful declaration.

# 14

# Integrity

*Real integrity is doing the right thing,*

*knowing that nobody's going to know*

*whether you did it or not.*

—OPRAH WINFREY

**To fully realize your vision you must *unite* liberation and manifestation. You've discovered creative/compassionate space and in this chapter you become skillful and strategic about exactly how to live into it. You also learn that when you *unite* with integrity it leads to samadhi (total immersion into your true nature) and dharma (your ultimate path).**

I was ambushed into becoming an entrepreneur. I'd like to say I walked into the business section of my local bookstore, bought several titles, spent months coming up with a twenty-year business model, and then dazzled a bunch of international financiers who handed me the keys to my studio. There are two problems with this scenario. One, unless Joan Didion starts writing how-to business books, you're not going to find me in the business section. Two, I had my yoga mat pulled out from under me before I could even get to the bookstore.

Let me explain.

After completing my training at the little local studio, I ended up teaching there for four years. Then, when sweeping administrative changes made it impossible for me to stay, I had only three weeks to get something going. That's not a typo—I only had three weeks. I didn't have a vision of my own place—name on the door, flashy logo, and merchandising. All I knew was that I had to make a brave move, pretty much yesterday. So just like that, I opened U Studio Yoga in Los Angeles, and ran it for nine years (that's about one hundred years anywhere else). It was named for the commUnity that built it with me in record-breaking time. Whether it was the lawyer who negotiated the deal, the architect who helped with the demolition, my father who put money toward my effort, or the unbelievably dedicated students who came with me, something extraordinary happened during our term there that I'd never known before. By the time we closed we'd seen each other through a wide variety of choices.

"It almost seems like those police helicopters are looking for one of us," I joked as we began to assemble for class one evening in our nest on the fifth floor of an art deco building. The bright lights bounced off the studio walls and around the surrounding streets, and the noise became deafening. In LA we've become so used to this kind of show we are not so easily impressed anymore. Road closures and police chases are as common as facelifts and boob jobs. It's just another moment when we feel like a cliché.

Then, one of us noticed a more colorful light display that seemed to be coming from the street. When we looked out our beautiful ten-foot windows to Wilshire below, we noticed the SWAT team, LAPD, and a sea of fire engines surrounding the building.

*That* got our attention.

More police could be heard on their way, and we caught word that no one was allowed in or out of the building. Many thoughts ran through my mind. What was I supposed to do? How could I keep my students from freaking out? And most importantly, how does a criminal on the lam end up in a Miracle Mile commercial building known more for its incredible architecture than as a haven for lawbreakers? The universe just shrugged its shoulders and pretended it didn't know what I was talking about.

Fifteen minutes (which felt like fifty) later, we noticed the backup leaving, and the SWAT members leaning up against their cars. A group of late students entered the room with the full story. The man the SWAT team had been pursuing had leapt to his death off the top of our building. We were safe, but things felt weird. There are a lot of awkward choices we're asked to make in life. For me, this was one of the creepier ones. Was it appropriate to teach the class now? Was it all the more necessary, or was it totally irresponsible?

After weighing my options, I opted to teach the class after all. As we left the building under the protective shield of our peaceful savasana, we passed the county coroner who was leaving, and a film crew arriving to prep for the car commercial they were shooting the next morning. The troubled man had died, but the "show must go on" LA stereotype was still alive and kicking.

All of this got me thinking about the choices we make and how they affect our lives. Yes, some choices come with a colorful backdrop and dramatic story like this one, but most are pretty innocuous and vanilla. We make silly little choices all the time: which pair of underwear to wear, whether to do single or double pigeon as our hip opener, what to download on iTunes, whether to follow someone on social media or not. Strung together, however, these choices actually determine the path of our lives.

If these seemingly insignificant moments are adding up to prodigious intervals, we want to ensure that they are heading us in the right direction. We need to pause, get clear, and use viveka (discernment) to remember the big picture our labyrinth of choices is designing.

How do we turn these teeny little puzzle pieces into the beautiful picture we want them to be? Our individual yoga practice is referred to as our yoga sadhana. It is unique to each of us, even though it is part of a larger system. Within our sadhana, we make practical choices about what we are and aren't willing to do. We calculate what will best serve us body and mind. If we decide to go too deeply into a pose like hanumanasana (vertical splits) without coming to that conclusion intuitively, we run the risk of injury. If we phone the whole thing in, we are not challenging ourselves to our potential, and wonder why there's been no change or inspiration. When we pay close attention, we find balance and we stay away from the precarious edges of extremes.

Dharma is to our life as sadhana is to our practice. It's our unique, personalized search for a more ethical way of living; it's our way of steering the ship even when the currents challenge or confuse our direction. Described by some as "cultivating right behavior" or "our religious duty," it is our path toward moral values. But morals can be tricky and susceptible to change depending on cultural circumstances and where we live. Not to mention that the word *religion* makes some of us more than a little bit uneasy. So let's break things down to their roots. *Relegere*, the Latin root for religion, means "to be aware." Dharma is the attempt to be fully aware and thoughtful in a universally responsible way. It's the lighthouse that guides our choices through the fog toward something higher and greater, whether we refer to that as God or someone or something else.

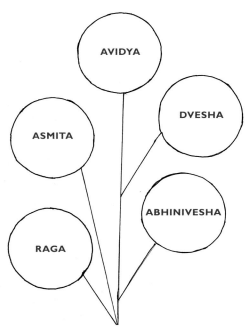

In Patanjali's *Yoga Sutras* as well as in Buddhist philosophy, *kleshas* translate as hindrances or obstacles. There are five of them, and you might call them behavioral bullrings we want to stay out of in order to follow the light of our dharma.

The first, avidya, is the King Klesha under which all other kleshas fall. It's commonly defined as ignorance. "Vid" relates to seeing, and connotes a misconception of reality. Avidya is the inability to access the Four Cs of our moral compass and to discern what does and doesn't matter when it comes to aligning with our integrity.

Our second klesha, dvesha, is avoidance of something we don't find pleasing. It's a reaction that keeps us ruminating in our aversion to something that's been challenging in the past, without seeing it as an opportunity for What's In the Way Is the Way. Dvesha is the spokesperson for "I can't/don't do that," and if we buy what dvesha's selling there will be no **Possibility**—be that pose, plan, or progress.

Whereas dvesha is avoiding that which we feel is unpleasant, raga is the desire to repeat things that feel good. Like limiting ourselves to only the poses we think we're good at, chasing the same feel-good-instant-gratification is narrow repetition that limits personal growth. Think too many cookies without the nourishment of an actual meal.

Our fourth klesha, asmita, means ego. All of us need a strong enough self-identity to operate in the world in which we live—we function as parents, partners, friends, employees, et cetera. But false perception or misrepresentation of our ego can take us off our dharmic path. We get tangled up in self-aggrandizing neediness or Val-you-less despair, to the extent that we lose sight of the truth. These spinning misconceptions keep us stuck in the false perceptions of our head and unable to access the intuitive heart of our integrity and dharma.

Lastly, abhinivesha means "clinging to life," which seems odd to consider as a hindrance, because instinctually survival is part of being alive. Right? I totally get that this is a super uncomfortable klesha to talk about . . . for me too. Very few things are guaranteed in this lifetime, but the fact that we will die is one of them. To me abhinivesha is the ultimate motivation to "do all of it," Become Bendy, see What's In the Way Is the Way, and begin again to create a Four C-able moment right now . . . because we won't be here forever. Our dharma is part of a divine spark within us that never dies. Whether you consider that legacy or spirit, connecting to what poet/philosopher David Whyte calls "the shape of your own absence" will allow you not to run from the fear of death, but to see it as the preeminent reason to live fully—as a transcendent reason to be planted instead of buried.

When we make our decisions from a more elevated state of consciousness instead of from knee-jerk reactions (see also: impatience, greed, carelessness, bozo in a bullring) we start to string together some beautiful potentials. We begin to take responsibility for our choices and therefore for the shape of our lives. The tiny puzzle pieces create a mosaic that feels genuine, attentive, extraordinary, and kind. Even without the SWAT team assembled below, we find ourselves awakened to the notion of doing the right thing.

Your savasanas, breathing, meditation, "pay close attention," and yoga practices are providing you with palpable examples of this mindful reflection. Our progression has brought you to a potent place where you are able to translate this mindful response vs. reaction from your mat to your life. To fully integrate body, mind and spirit is to find *samadhi* (our true nature). To *unite* with samadhi is to align holistically with our integrity.

**noun: *integrity***

1.  the quality of being honest and having strong moral principles; moral uprightness.

2.  the state of being whole and undivided.

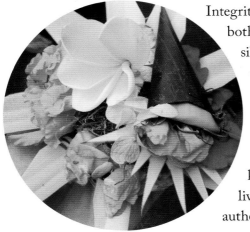

Integrity asks us to be accountable for how we're showing up both for ourselves and for those around us—to be responsible for what we're putting into our bodies and minds as well as what we're putting out into the world. That includes not only our actions but also our words. Even gossip and drama can pollute our environment. As the late Maya Angelou said, they can "climb into the woodwork, into the furniture and the next thing you know they're on your skin." Defining your choices and living with compassion and integrity will lead to your authentic path—your dharma.

## ON YOUR MAT

Becoming Bendy enough to uncover our dharma is evidence that we're transforming into beginners armed with Four Cs, Practice Makes Progress, and Val-you. Each time we fold into ourselves on our mat, we're reminded of the stretching we're doing that reaches far beyond its borders. The discomfort we feel in our apprehensive muscles and tricky-to-focus minds are the same What's In the Way Is the Way opportunities we're folding into our lives one breath at a time. Body/mind/spirit is no longer a catchphrase or secret esoteric code out there somewhere that we can't access—we're soaking in it. We're living "how you do your yoga is how you do your life."

Mr. Iyengar (the father of Iyengar yoga) spoke about "good pain." It's the dull roar of finding new strength and flexibility as we practice—not to be confused with the electrical pain that is a warning of injury otherwise known as "bad pain." We develop an intimate relationship with good pain in our yoga practice. You might say it's where viveka (staying out of the bullring) and "pay close attention" meet. In fact, these sensations are really what asana is about. We use them to cross over into new thresholds in our bodies and minds. Like any intimate relationship, it's full of nuance and subtlety. Thoughtless or neglectful actions can lead to unfortunate outcomes. If we're not careful, competing, spacing out, pushing too far, or not really trying can litter the nuance. Take twists as an example. The goal is not to become a human corkscrew. We are wringing deeply into muscles and our spine, staying within the integrity of "good pain" while avoiding the avidya of "bad pain."

Let's use twisting anjaneyasana (low lunge) as an example. I'd like you to do a few of our surya namaskar As first, so that you're warm, pre-windup. Refer back to page 42 if you need a refresher and don't forget @OM as an option for these. Make sure you read through the exercise below before heading back in to attempt it.

After your surya namaskar As, find child's pose and S.T.O.P. to S.T.A.R.T. Try to narrow your breath down to in and out through your nose, and scrape the breath against the back of your throat to create the texture and sound of ujjayi breathing. Stay for five or six full cycles and find the inward turn of pratyahara. Then curl your toes under and lift your hips up and back for down dog.

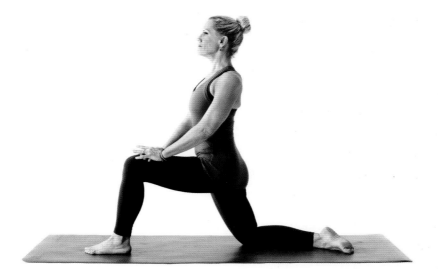

As a departure from our samskara (habit) of always starting with our right side, I'm going to have you step your left foot forward first from down dog into a low lunge with your right knee down on the ground behind you.

Be sure to use padding—a blanket, towel or cushion of some sort—if your right knee is sensitive. Curling your back toes under can help alleviate stress to that back knee here too. Zero "bad pain" is to be endured.

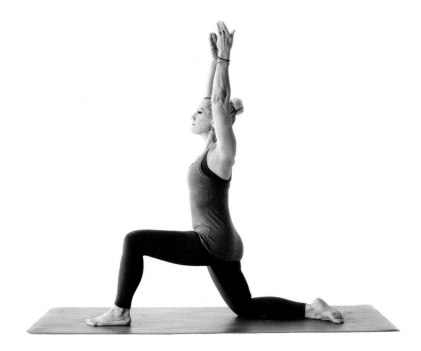

**Place your hands on your front thigh for support. Feel a sense of deep roots into the ground, noticing your body's connection to the earth. Each exhale adds to this foundation. Lengthen your tailbone toward the ground and the top of your head to the sky, pressing gently into your hands on top of your left thigh for stability while you adventure into your spine. Find tadasana in your torso as you reach both arms overhead. Incline your pinky fingers toward each other and your thumbs apart, finding external rotation at the shoulder joint.**

Notice that the architecture of this alignment creates freedom and space in your neck and shoulders without you forcing anything anywhere. Feel your trunk as 360 degrees— your front, back, and side ribs lifting spaciously off your pelvis as you grow incrementally taller with every inhale.

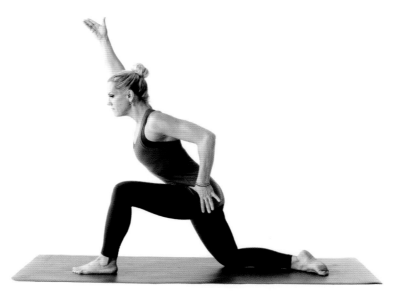

Keeping as much length in your torso as you can, take your left thumb into your left hip crease. Draw that left hip back and down as if it were interested in visiting your right heel. Still reaching your right arm up to the sky, excavate space between the ribs and pelvis on both sides of your waist and back body.

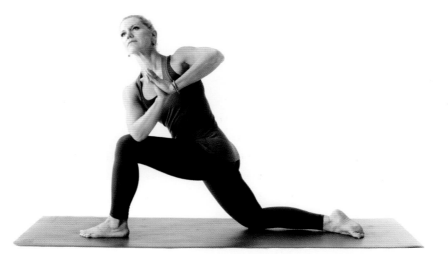

Hinge at your hips and snuggle your right elbow to the outside of your left thigh. Press into your left hand to create extension, almost as if encouraging a little bit of a cobra in your midback where your shoulder blades attach to your spine. Bring your hands into a prayer in front of your middle chest.

At the bottom of each exhale, stay empty and use the leverage of your prayer like a little loving nudge to go just a bit deeper into your twist until you brush up against your edge. Allow the appropriate intensity to remain—neither crossing the line into punishment nor backing off too far for Practice Makes Progress to occur. The more you elongate your spine, the more room there is to rotate your twist when you exhale. You're going to stay here for six full cycles of breath.

Instead of being preoccupied with variations in this twist (lifting up your back knee, extending your bottom arm toward the ground and top arm to the sky, snuggling your bottom shoulder underneath your front thigh and interlacing your hands behind your back in a bind), remain with your hands at your heart, back knee on the floor, and pay close attention. Remember that vinyasa means breath guiding the movement and placing with special and deliberate care. Variations in poses are like the leaves on a tree. They come and go with seasons and the weather. Our roots and our trunk are foundational and connect us consistently to the branches of our practice that matter most—to the integrity of our Eight Limbs instead of the bullring of our Five Kleshas.

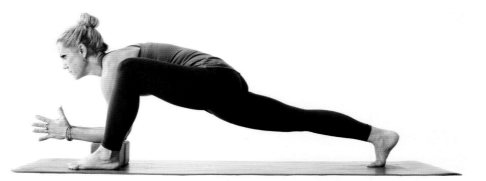

**Unwind out of your twist carefully, and place both hands onto the ground on the inside of your left foot. You're going to pause here for a moment in a variation of humble warrior.**

Perhaps you bring your forearms to the ground or a block for this. A few of you might even curl your back toes under and take the back knee off your mat. Be humble, not desperate, as you meet yourself where you are. Feel sthira (steadiness)/sukham (ease) and a savasana breeze. When you're open to being humbled it is extraordinary evidence that you are on the path—whether that's in your lunge or in your life. Steep in all the goodness of this posture for a full minute (or longer if you'd like).

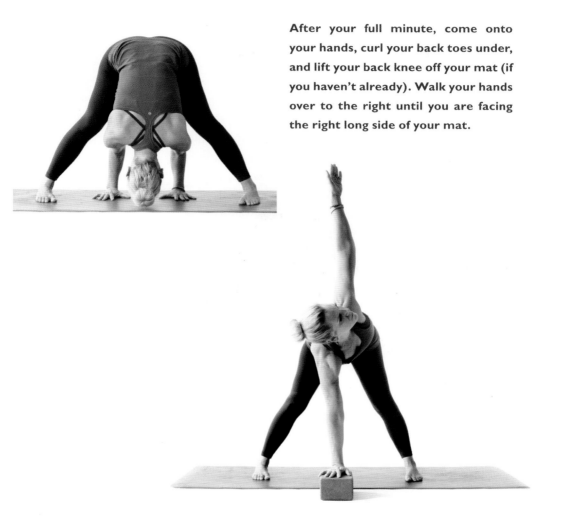

**After your full minute, come onto your hands, curl your back toes under, and lift your back knee off your mat (if you haven't already). Walk your hands over to the right until you are facing the right long side of your mat.**

**Line up the edges of your feet with the short edges of your mat and tone your legs toward straight without locking them into hyperextension. Enjoy a few moments here. Then bring your torso parallel to the ground. Place your right hand on the ground or a block directly underneath your face, and bring your left hand to your low belly as you did on your fingertips, hands, and knees in our core work earlier. Feel the uddiyana bandha (light corseting of your belly toward your spine) under that left hand acting as support. Then bring that left hand onto your low back.**

Turn your chest open to the left, twisting in this new configuration like you did in your low lunge a few moments ago. Catch a whiff of a cobra backbend in your midback as opposed to rounding there, and see if your neck is struggling to steal the spotlight by working way too hard. Extend your left arm up to the sky (or keep it on your low back if this is enough). Linger for six full cycles of breath, then carefully unwind both hands to the ground.

Pause here in a contemplative forward fold with your hands on blocks, your shins, or ankles, or on the ground (prasarita padottanasana A) . Maybe you even interlace your hands behind your back (prasarita padottanasana C). Holding a strap or towel between your hands will afford you more space to play with. Bask in a full-minute release here.

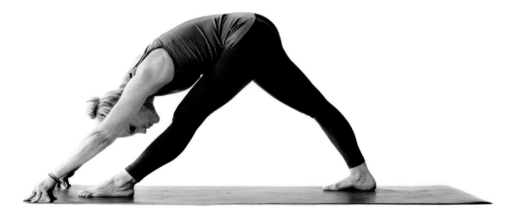

**From your prasarita forward fold, walk both hands to the left, wandering back the way you came in. Keeping this wide space between your straight front and back legs, frame your left foot with your fingertips on either side for a forward fold stretch in pyramid pose (parsvotanansa).**

Inch your left foot to the left a little bit to provide more sideways space here. Blocks under your hands will bring the ground up to you if that's helpful. Wandering farther forward or back with your hands might give you a bit more stretch sensation if that's what you're looking for.

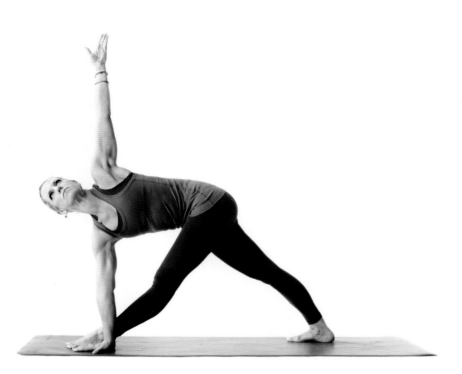

**Take your left thumb into your left hip crease, like you did in your low lunge. Finding a light lift to your low belly (uddiyana bandha), reach your torso parallel to the ground (much as you did facing the long edge of your mat a minute ago). Extend your right arm out in front, toward the front of your mat, creating space on both sides of the waist—pulling your left hip back in contrast to those right fingers reaching forward. Then place your right hand on the inside (for most of us) or possibly the outside of your left foot (a block would be excellent here) and your left hand on your low back. Begin to rotate your chest to the left, twisting as you have in the previous two poses.**

Float your left arm up to the sky (or let it remain on your low back if that works best right now). Remain for six cycles of breath, then gently unwind and step back into downward facing dog.

Take side two of this little sequence either translating the above to your right side, or using @OM. Then snuggle into a child's pose.

Be sure to take a few moments to visit your tree and **Possibility Pose**.

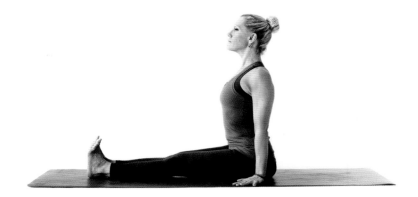

Then make your way to a seated position, legs straight out in front of you (dandasana).

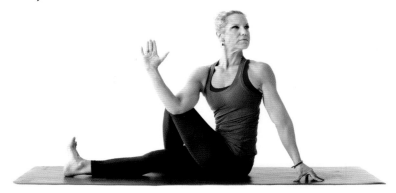

Bend your left knee and step that foot onto the floor to the outside of your right thigh.

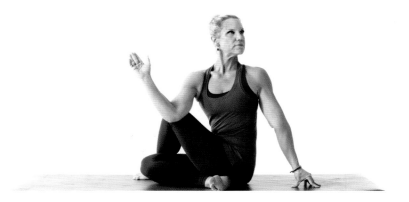

Optionally, bend your right knee, bringing your right heel toward your left butt-cheek (yes, I said butt-cheek).

Take your left hand to the ground behind you and your right arm up to the sky. Either hug your left knee with your right arm, or take the right triceps to the outside of your left thigh for a twist (ardha matsyendrasana). Sitting on a block or blanket and even using a block beneath the hand behind you can be wonderfully beneficial. The same principles apply to this twist as the others. Inhale length—exhale loving nudge to guide you in a bit deeper. Think elegant and spacious vs. curlicue aggression. Try to remain here for ten full cycles of breath. Then carefully unwind and take side two.

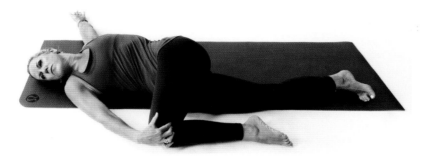

**Once you've completed both sides, lie down onto your back and hug your left knee into your chest. Take your left arm straight out to the side, or into a cactus shape. Cross your left knee all the way over your body to rest on the floor on the right side of you for a supine twist.**

If it doesn't reach all the way to the floor don't worry. It might be nice to rest that knee on your block, or just let it hover for now. Still no "bad pain" in the mix . . . right? It can be helpful to skooch your hips a little to the left so that you are on the outside of your right hip, creating a little bit more space for your twist. Perhaps using your right hand gently on your left thigh feels like some nice encouragement too. Stay here five to six cycles of breath before you gently unwind and take the second side. Once finished with both supine sides, delight in a five-minute savasana. Set your timer if you're not using @OM.

The physical benefits of twisting our bodies helps to free us from atrophy. As we fine-tune the actions of the pose we enhance these benefits. Because it is a work in progress, our idea of a goal is ever evolving and truly holistic. As you deconstruct your personal growth this way on your mat, you carry it with you out into the world. As tempting as a quick fix can be, it's ultimately limited and even stifling. You have to move through your share of good pain to get to the good gain. This is ideal preparation for the twists and

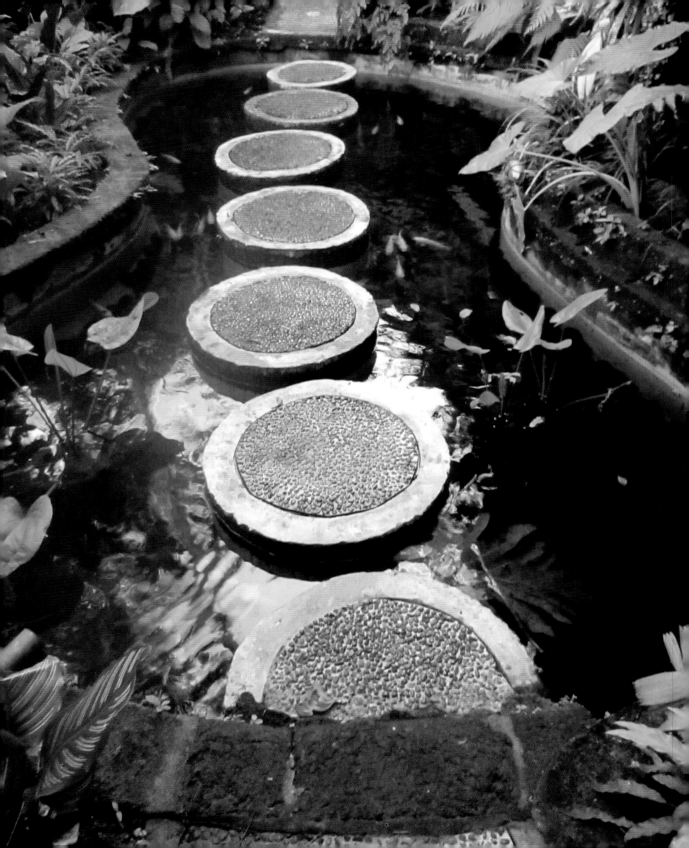

turns you'll inevitably experience along your way as you step deeper into integrity and dharma **On Your OM.**

## ON YOUR OM

There's no single word in Western languages that translates the definition of dharma: right way of living, ultimate path come close. Its root, *dhri*, means to support or hold. You might say dharma is the expansive container in which your compassion, creativity, and integrity want to live. And it consists of the discoveries you've made in the pages of this book. But like many of the deceivingly simple poses we've visited here together, dharma too can feel elusive when it's our turn to integrate it into our lives.

I believe a sense of personal purpose is the gateway that transitions dharma from outside concept to accessible path.

Certainly that's been my experience. Purpose is defined as our reason for doing something—our motivation, intent, justification, and design. Some people call it our personal legend or legacy. To me, purpose is the omnipresent pulse at the heart of our fully realized lives. When I uncovered my purpose, it led me to my dharma.

So how do we get in touch with our purpose? First by being, as Paulo Coelho said, "a person who is proud to be a pilgrim, and who's trying to honor his journey." Which is exactly what you and I are up to.

There are three specific questions that helped me get clear in terms of purpose:

1.   What do you love to do?

2.   Who or what do you do it for?

3.   What is it that shifts, changes, or transforms for you as a result? For others? For the world?

When I was a singer/songwriter my answer for "What do you love to do?" was music. But when it came to "Who or what do you do it for?," I was at a loss. "What shifts or transforms for you as a result?" was even murkier. In fact, I was so busy competing when it came to making music that I'd locked myself out of my laboratory and into a miserable spin cycle of comparison insecurity. But, What's In the Way Is the Way . . .

Music alone was neither my purpose nor my dharma, but it was a stepping-stone toward discovering both. Skills I acquired translated perfectly into teaching yoga —guiding a room full of people with my voice, composing a sequence lyrically and intuitively like songwriting, even curating musical playlists for my classes. Music was, and continues to be, a supporting section in my full life's symphony. There are people like Joni Mitchell whose purpose and dharma are, in fact, music—they'd have no problem answering questions two and three. My ultimate purpose lay elsewhere. My willingness to "do all of it"—to be a vulnerable beginner, ready to learn, bend, and grow—revealed to me an extraordinary personal pilgrimage. One I will spend the rest of my life trying to honor. When it comes to teaching yoga, I know exactly who and what I am doing it for. I do it for you. And the shifts, changes, and transformations I witness blow my mind —sure, within myself, but even more so within all of you. You give me purpose. Thank you.

I bet, as you continue to pay close attention both on your mat and off, you will start to recognize your music—the rich voices of seemingly disparate experiences that crescendo in concert with your purpose and dharma.

Earlier I had you come up with solutions for your **Stuckat List**—in other words, for what you don't want. Remember? You turned your drive time into inspired time. Now I'm going to ask you to find the same for your list of what you *do* want. What's exciting is that the tools you've accrued, including the less-than-linear **On Your OM** exercises from our last chapter, will inspire the courageous creativity and honest, open heart you need to start to transform **Stuckat List** into **Close to OM**.

Grab your notebook.

Set it off to the side for a moment and S.T.O.P. to S.T.A.R.T. Take a five-minute seated meditation. Give yourself conscious space to shift from reaction to response right off the bat. Let your breath land you in your body and allow your attention to turn inward (pratyahara). By taking innovative initiative, you're announcing to yourself and to the world that you're ready to move forward. You're declaring that you will do so with compassion, show up with integrity, and be fully accountable for the choices you make. Think of this as skillful and strategic action in the direction of your purpose and dharma.

Start with a ten-year vision. Build upon the letter you wrote and sent to yourself in our From Your Head to Your Heart chapter. Become even more detailed as you describe how these wants on your list have manifested ten years from now. Where are you living?

What are the smells, the sounds, the tastes? What's on your bedside table? Who's with you? Think of this as coming up with an address to enter into your GPS. Even if you end up living a few doors down, you now have a vision of where you're going. Write it all down. You'll be adding to it in the future.

Move to five years from now. How much of your ten-year vision has been realized, and what does that look like? If your vision was to open a bed-and-breakfast in Costa Rica, what steps have you taken to get there? Have you had experience working in the hospitality business? Do you know how to manage a property? Have you learned to speak Spanish? Are you talking to investors or do you have your own capital? Do you know anything about Costa Rica? Have you ever even been there to visit? Are there times when you feel tension rise up in your body as you think about this? Can you breathe your way back to clarity and calm? Can you turn every moment into an opportunity to learn? Are you able to stay with your solution instead of becoming distracted or tangled up in competition or expectation? Can you allow mistakes to be insightful blessings? Are you able to listen to your heart as well as your head?

And finally, at this very moment, what are you doing toward your vision? You now have the long view and the tools to become wildly creative, proactive, and productive! Remind yourself that abhyasa (persevering practice) and vairagya (surrender) are crucial. We are invested in our process and not locked into a specific end result. An expansive view is just that—ripe with the fluidity of possibility.

Take a Spanish class. Save money and arrange your schedule so you can visit Costa Rica by the end of the year. By going, you might discover that you'd rather open your B&B in Colorado, but you can't know that until you create space for yourself to learn. And if you end up in Colorado it's not because you've failed. It's because you were willing to let life be a laboratory instead of a contest. Remember, in a laboratory there's no winning or losing, no success or failure, there's just observing, information, and inspiration. Maybe you start to work at a hotel and realize it's not what you thought it would be. But while you're there you fall in love with being in the kitchen and see that your dharma is more farm-to-table than it is general manager. Had you not taken action and taken the job, you'd have missed an opportunity that you hadn't even been able to see yet. You are "doing all of it." You are on the path. You have your finger on the pulse of your purposeful pilgrimage.

# 15

# Connection

*The need for connection and community is primal, as fundamental as the need for air, water and food.*

—DR. DEAN ORNISH

**In this chapter you learn that connection, community, and purpose are key to living into your richest capacity and santosha (a deep-seated sense of contentment). To *unite* is to turn inward ultimately so that you can reach out.**

The mission to create a life of compassion, purpose, connection, and integrity is ongoing. And we need only look to the Upanishads written nearly 1,500 years ago to see that we've been contemplating this for a while:

*Watch your thoughts; they become words*
*Watch your words; they become actions*
*Watch your actions; they become habits*
*Watch your habits; they become character*
*Watch your character; for it becomes your destiny*

Purusha is pure consciousness, supreme intelligence, eternal soul, our highest Self. It is our individual voice in an infinite choir. It's the relationship between purusha and the prakriti we spoke of back in chapter 5 that helps us evolve toward understanding. Prakriti is all the stuff our soul bumps up against while we're here on earth. It is what Sri Swami Satchidananda calls our "universe-ity."

Yoga is like an archeological dig to uncover our true Self. It liberates us and reminds us that we are citizens of the world. Stretching and enriching our interior landscape makes us more tuned in to our interconnectedness to everything and everyone else. Our yoga mats are magic carpets to look into our lives and to see the world. Or as Socrates put it, "Let him who would move the world first move himself." When we feel inspired, fulfilled, and alive we want others to *awaken*, *tranform*, and *unite* with us.

When I heard Kate Braestrup's story on *On Being* while I was hiking, I took another loop around the canyon to catch her entire interview. She's a chaplain in Maine who accompanies the game wardens on search and rescue missions that often involve loss and disaster: people driving off the side of a snow-covered road, or going missing in the wild. Because she lost her own husband unexpectedly in an instant, she knows how important it is to have people around us as we face life's challenges. Time and time again, she sees the power and beauty of people showing up for one another during a time of need, the juxtaposition of crisis and compassion. To use her words: "The question isn't whether we're going to have to do hard, awful things, because we are—we all are. The question is whether we have to do them alone. There is this sense of a community that will hold us."

In my classroom, we witness each other's lives too. We see each other through the down economy, watch the beautiful pregnant bellies among us turn into miraculous new extended family members. Broken hearts are comforted and new exciting jobs celebrated. We're not in the wilderness of Maine, we're in the jungle of the city, and I am no chaplain. But human stories do not adhere to zip codes or territories. They belong to us all. To share them with each other is to hold each other close.

I think we all need a safe place to smooth out our crumpled lives, a place where we can reveal our warts and wrinkles and not feel judged. And since we are certainly smoothing out our buckled bodies and minds with our yoga, it is a natural conduit to reach out to one another for connection and community.

Faith can be hard to find on our own. We fumble in our darkness, and then someone holds up a flashlight to help us find our way. When someone else believes in us, we begin to believe in ourselves—and before you know it, we are holding up the flashlight for someone else. We are *all* warriors with the power to illuminate one another, and when we do we are as beautiful as the stars in the sky.

I'm grateful for the brave, inspiring warriors who grace my path. Here are a few of the stories they've allowed me to share with you. I cannot wait to hear your stories too!

## WARRIOR I

When she came on retreat to Mexico, Sherry was terrified of the bugs, the food, the accommodations (which were luxury), and the sun. While everyone else was raving about the place, splashing in the surf, and sipping hibiscus water, she found nothing acceptable. It was six days of misery in paradise.

Never would I have foreseen what she proved capable of two years later.

After her boyfriend proposed with the only size diamond she would allow, they were married and had a beautiful baby boy. When she was three months pregnant with her second child, doctors discovered stage-four breast cancer. It was strongly recommended that she abort the baby, as they had to do extreme chemo and radical treatment. She refused and bravely entered uncharted waters, receiving the treatments while the baby grew inside her.

During this time she would often cyber-chat with me. She was not able to physically practice, but the yoga she was doing, breathing through this unbelievable situation, was far more sophisticated than I could ever teach. She, who'd not been particularly focused on her mat, was unwavering on this battlefield. She wanted to find the deeper aspects of her yoga, the "spiritual" ones, and we gently wandered through what that might mean to her.

Miracles can be challenging to reconcile. The baby was born healthy and she is cancer-free. She is grateful, but true to form, she is not afraid to point to what is unsatisfactory. I learned from Sherry that there is a warrior in all of us, even those of us who would appear to need to outsource such bravery. We don't know what we are capable of until we are challenged to the limit. Sherry reminded me that inspiration is not precious, with the string section swelling and the lighting just so. It is human, and impatient, and still true to who it always was.

## WARRIOR 2

Louisa's limbs were twisted by muscular dystrophy. She wandered in and started to set up. I was concerned—mine is a rigorous class, and I wanted to protect her without making a spectacle. It is a line every teacher walks with any new student, but her circumstances had me feeling all the more conflicted about how hands on or off I should be.

To my surprise, I marveled at her customized poses, and how well she knew herself. Then, when she called me over to spot her in a headstand, something I would not have imagined her attempting, I realized something. She was more aware of what her limitations *were* than most of us, but she was also more aware of what they *weren't*. She was spectacular, explaining to me that because her right arm couldn't bend correctly, she would need me to adjust my stance to best support her. She didn't need my counsel— what she needed was for me to find the faith that she already had.

## WARRIOR 3

A statuesque blonde and a shorter, older-than-her screenwriter husband are not uncommon in Los Angeles. When I arrived at the door for their first private session, Seth and Elaine both had cigarettes in their hands. "You're probably going to need to put those out before we get started," I remember myself saying. They were fun and funny and we practiced outside next to their babbling brook.

But things were not all that they seemed.

Checks started bouncing, and hushed cash was handed to me by the blonde in secret. There was evidence of fighting, and the drama began to seep into our sessions and scheduling. After a while I'd stop hearing from them all together. This became a pattern that continued over a few years, and they moved several times as well.

Then, after months of not hearing a thing, Seth found me and wanted to practice on his own. They were divorcing; he was devastated and felt deceived. It seems the money she was supposedly using for their taxes and bills had ended up financing her drug habit instead.

Heartbroken and broke, he crawled back onto his mat one more time looking for some answers. It was slow going at first. He spent a lot of time talking about her during the hip openers. Stories and recollections tended to repeat. But little by little he found his breath again. I pressed him to come to the group classes because I knew that community was the missing piece this time around. I look at him often in the front row of a crowded class now, enjoying his tribe and beaming. Somewhere along the way he stopped smoking too.

Yes, we are looking for someone to hear us, but we want a place to *belong* too . . . a place where we can shine with the other lights on the tree—a tree with deep roots and wide branches.

## ON YOUR MAT

Santosha is a profound sense of contentment for what is, even as we move toward improvement. It's a universal connection to underlying joy, despite tough and trying times. Santosha asks us to welcome the realities of life as we accede to our dharmic path and highest purpose. Santosha helps to keep us out of the emotional bullring so we can live into What's In the Way Is the Way. On our mat, santosha is where the integrity of our mountain and the surrender of our savasana coexist. Where we learn to listen to the ubiquitous insight within the pose instead of imposing restless judgment or expectation from outside.

Restorative postures cultivate santosha within our personal fabric. And when we *unite* with our own sense of contentment, we can't wait to wear and extend it out into the world. One important thing to understand about restoratives is that gravity does the work—not you. In fact, your biggest challenge will be to relinquish your incessant doing and simply be. Allow every exhale to bring you a little closer to savasana as tranquility takes the wheel. Use your silent "'let' on the inhale, 'go' on the exhale" mantra.

For many of us who enjoy the rigors of vinyasa-style flow, the "simply be" element of restorative practice kicks up a lot of fidgety, agitated dust. If you're like me, you may catch a glimpse of just how attached you are to accomplishment. Don't scold yourself. It's not terrible for us to aspire to do things. Just think back to what you've learned about your nervous system. When you're desperate to keep your foot on the stress-response gas pedal, opt for applying the relaxation-response brake instead. Lean into santosha, and believe with every breath that your Val-you is innate and to be celebrated, not the result of punishing reproach or performance. As time with our tree and **Possibility Pose** has proven, if we're going to "do all of it," there has to be effort *and* surrender—sthira sukham asanam (steady and sweet practice). It's the only way we'll stay planted and not buried.

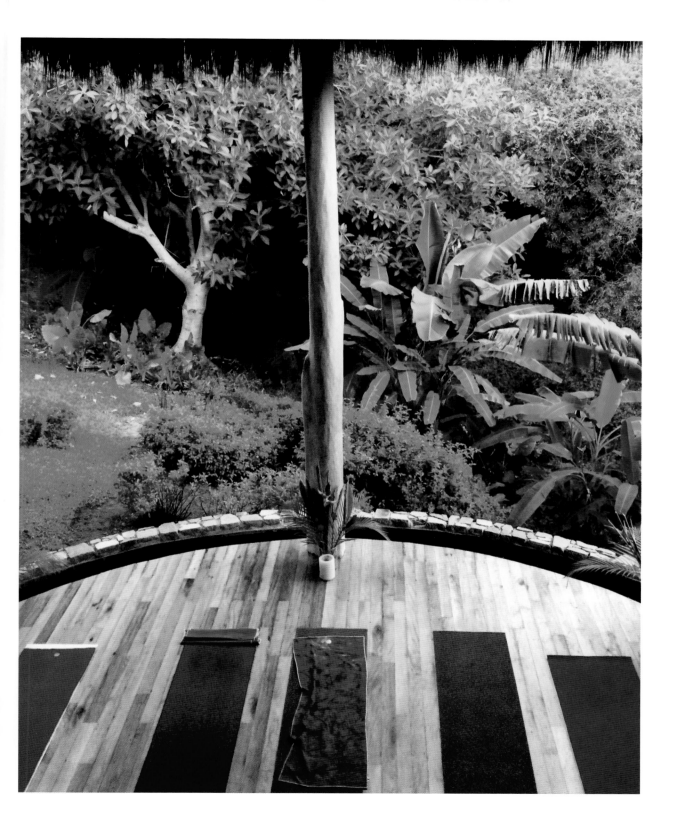

For this restorative sequence, you're going to use some props. Since not all of you have a yoga studio selection of blocks or bolsters lying around, I'm going to offer up some household alternatives. I often use the cushions from a couch or chair when I need props for a private client or when I'm traveling. You can also stack two firm pillows on top of one another for what we're going to do. It's actually pretty fun to be inventive. When I reference bolster, it will mean whatever you've designated as your prop. I've seen anything from a piece of carry-on luggage to a giant kid's teddy bear in my time. Beware of sharp edges or pointy barbs like zippers—oh, and Lego building sets won't work . . . I speak from experience. You'll want a couple of big towels or small blankets handy too. Remember to read through below before jumping in and actually doing it, so you get the lay of the land first. (We will omit our tree and **Possibility Pose** from this progression, but you will find options for ways to combine this restorative practice with other postures in appendix 1.)

Let's start in a cross-legged seat for a five-minute meditation. I love to sit on at least one of my pillows, or upon my cushion/bolster. The rule of thumb here is that if your knees are higher than your hips when you're cross-legged, you'll want to elevate your seat on something. Five minutes can feel like five hours if you're miserable, so make your perch a balance of easeful and interesting. You'll S.T.O.P. to S.T.A.R.T. and weave in your ABCs. You don't need to add ujjayi for restoratives. Just breathe deeply through your nose instead of your mouth. See if you can already sense santosha trickling in. Use your timer or @OM.

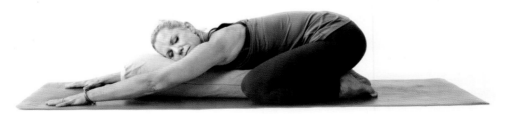

**Once you're done with your meditation, situate your bolster or stacked pillows for a supported child's pose. It can be pretty heavenly to roll up a big towel or a small blanket and put it between your hips and your heels. Let your big toes touch and allow enough room between your knees to slide in your support. Feel the rise and fall of your breath against your bolster—a juicy wide inhale and softening exhale. Turn your head to one side and enjoy three minutes here.**

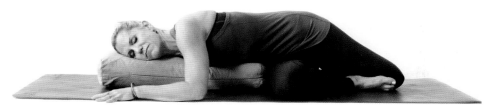

**Keep your bolster where it is, but resituate yourself so that your right hip is resting against the short edge. Your butt's on the ground, but it looks as if you are riding sidesaddle. Lie out over your bolster on your right side. Extend your right arm and use it as if it were a pillow on top of your cushion. Take a few breaths here to appreciate the space that you are creating along your side body and in your spine. Still sidesaddle, support yourself with your hands on either side of your bolster, turning your chest and torso toward your cushion. Lower down onto your support in this new position, keeping your head facing the same direction as your knees. If you scissor your top leg back behind you, toward the left a bit, you may feel a little more *oomph* to your twist. You're also welcome to turn your head to face to the right (away from your knees). That's going to make things more intense on your neck. So be careful what you wish for.**

We are going to stay on this side for five minutes. Set your timer or use **@OM**.

Be sure to come out the same way you came in. Begin by turning your head the direction of your knees again if you've turned it away from them, and take a few breaths here. Linger with your right arm overhead. Then use your hands on, or to the sides of, your bolster to come upright and shift your sidesaddle the other direction. Left hip up against your cushion, lie out onto your left side, using your left arm now as an extended pillow. After a few moments here, turn your torso and chest to face the bolster. Lower down, head facing the same way that your knees are initially. If you'd like to adjust your top leg or turn your head to add intensity feel free. Enjoy five minutes on this side. Then slowly come out the way that you came in.

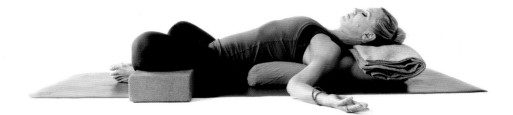

**You're now going to make your way into supta baddha konasana. Your bolster can stay where it is. Take one of your towels or blankets and fold it or roll it like you're making a little burrito for your head. Place it at the far end of your bolster as a pillow. Sit right in front of your bolster and lie back down on the support. Adjust your burrito under the back of your head but let your shoulders drape over your bolster, free of the burrito. Once you're situated, place the bottoms of your feet together with your knees out to the side. If this is tight, your knees and inner thighs might start to rebel during your stay, so have a couple of blocks, additional pillows, or rolled up towels or blankets nearby to slide under your thighs if you need them.**

This pose is one of my favorite things on the planet. It's the most amazing counterpose to how we slump at our computers and close down our hearts and hips throughout the day. Imagine your muscles as liquid, and let them drip down over your props, succumbing to gravity's caress. If any whispers of tension like our first exercise make their way into this restorative moment, know that you need only administer more love to untangle them. That might come from adding additional props, a longer exhale, or simply taking a moment to R.A.T. out (Recognize, Acknowledge, and Transform from chapter 7) anxious tendencies (samskara) and return them to peaceful renewal. Self-aware begets self-care. You will stay here for at least five minutes. Use your timer or @OM.

To come out of supta baddha konasana, first gently draw your knees together, using your hands on the outside of your thighs to assist. Pause, then roll to either side, coming carefully off your bolster and into fetal pose. When you're ready, use the strength of your arms to bring yourself up to sitting with your head the last thing up.

Make your way to a wall. We're going to take viparita karani. (Another of my favorite things.) Though this posture is often referenced as "legs up the wall" pose, the Sanskrit translates as viparita = inverted or reversed, and karani = making or doing. Viparita karani makes us reverse the actions and inverts the way in which we sit or stand all day. It is absolutely delicious, and the calming effects are palpable especially if you've been traveling, standing, walking, or running a lot. It feels like you're rinsing the swollen fatigue out of your legs, it supports and soothes your back, plus lying down tends to lower your heart rate and inspire your relaxation response. The Harvard Medical School even lists viparita karani (alongside supta baddha, konasana, child's pose, and savasana) as helpful for better sleep (http://www.health.harvard.edu/blog/8753-201512048753). Other benefits associated with viparita karani are relief from headaches and anxiety, and improved circulation. (If you have glaucoma or high blood pressure you'll want to be sensitive and not stay too long in this, or any inversion. Consult your doctor to be clear on your specific condition.)

You can do viparita karani with or without props. (You can even do viparita karani without a wall: from bridge pose (page 85) carefully slide a block, sturdy bolster, or folded blankets underneath your tailbone, then, sitting solidly on your prop, draw your knees into your chest and, as much as your hamstrings will allow, straighten your legs up to the sky.) I do it everywhere—seriously, when I'm traveling it's the first thing I do in my hotel room. I've put my legs up trees in London parks and on Mexican hillsides, the back of a chair in the Delhi airport, the side of a train when I had a whole row of seats to myself. I'm shameless. When you fly economy like I do for long stretches of time, viparita karani is the elephant-ankle/cabin-pressure antidote. But even just traveling through a typical day can call for some neutralizing, don't you think?

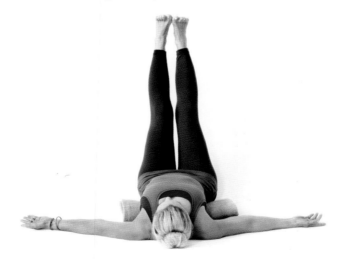

**To climb in, you'll sit sidesaddle with your right hip near the wall, much like you did at the front of your bolster a moment ago. Everybody's spacing is going to be a little bit different here. Tight hamstrings will factor in, as will lower back con-**

**cerns (which are often related to one another). You'll be able to maneuver once you're up there. From your sidesaddle seat, lean over onto your left elbow and swoop both legs up the wall. Once your legs are up, you can bend your knees and put your feet on the wall to lift your hips away from the ground and move closer to or farther from the wall.**

If you're interested in using props here, before you swoop up, place your bolster or a folded blanket in front of your wall with enough space for your butt to snuggle closer to the wall and your sacrum/lower back supported by the bolster. Think sit bones spilling off the bolster and toward the wall with a natural curvature in your lower back. Make sure this feels good in your body. For some people, placing the blanket under the sit bones without the curve to the lower spine is the answer. Play around with it a bit and see what works for you. You can adjust your blanket placement by bending your knees, putting your feet on your wall once you're up, lifting your hips, and carefully moving the blanket into place beneath you. You might also enjoy a folded blanket under your head. Then, once the porridge is just right, snuggle in for five minutes, using your timer or @OM.

I typically stay here for ten minutes. And I often use it as my savasana. There are also a few leg variations I enjoy sometimes. You can add supta baddha konasana legs here, placing the bottoms of your feet together, knees out to the side. Another really great option is straight legs out to the side in upvistha konasana.

To come out of viparita karani, bend your knees into your chest and gently push into the wall with your feet to come onto your side. Shift into a comfortable seat position and rest your back against the wall for a moment. You can sit on your bolster or blanket if you'd like. Perhaps our original cross-legged seat speaks to you here.

We're going to end with what's called a Metta meditation. Metta (*maitri* in Sanskrit) translates as loving-kindness. It connotes unconditional acceptance and friendship with oneself and an active interest in others. Full disclosure, I wasn't sure what I thought of this Metta business when I was first introduced to it, and it took me a moment to "get it." So if you wrestle with a little cynical pushback around this initially, know that I was skeptical too. But none of us really want to be too stoic or defensive to embrace loving-kindness, do we? Just let it wash over you and take what speaks to you right now; leave what doesn't. Personally, once it landed for me, it was huge. It's become a prominent flavor in my meditation gumbo and my touchstone for *unite*.

I'm going to give you the verbiage I use for my Metta meditation. There are many variations of these words out there, and you can also riff on them a bit and create your own. Myriad techniques for Metta abound for you to explore. For our purposes today, I'm using a truncated adaptation that I often visit at the end of my meditation or yoga practice.

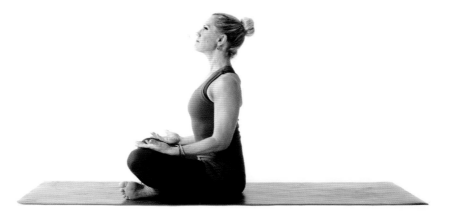

**You can stay here, seated cross-legged, perhaps with your back against the wall, or move to a sit in a chair or anywhere else that's comfortable. You're also welcome to remain with your legs up the wall in viparita karani for this. Another option is to lie on the ground in savasana. It's pretty great to experiment with all of these alternatives from time to time. I tend to swap them out depending on what I'm feeling that day.**

Once you're settled in, close your eyes and breathe into your ABCs. Take a moment to note the sounds inside and outside the room without commentary. Just observe. Feel yourself fully present to what is, not ruminating in the past or rehearsing for the future. Stay a full minute here.

We'll start our Metta as "I" and then expand it out to "we." Just as you've witnessed within the progression of this book, we start with our Self and ultimately reach out to one another. I highly recommend @OM for this, but feel free to read things over and then silently repeat this meditation on your own.

## METTA MEDITATION

*May I be happy*
*May I live my life with ease*
*May I be free from internal and external harm*
*May I love and accept myself completely—exactly as I am right now*
*May I be happy*

(Pause for five cycles of breath.)

*May we be happy*
*May we live our lives with ease*
*May we be free from internal and external harm*
*May we love and accept ourselves completely—exactly as we are right now*
*May we be happy*

You can repeat this as many or as few times as you like. Perhaps you stay seated for a few rounds and then take a classic (non-Metta-infused) savasana. I'd like for your ending meditation to be five minutes, whether that's all Metta or a combination of Metta and savasana. Let this be a sweet finish to your restorative practice. Marinate in the goodness you've uncovered by simply carving out the space to be thoughtful and caring in your own direction. Notice how much you want to spread the loving-kindness of Metta from "I" to "we" out in the world now too.

# ON YOUR OM

Since we're beginning to see ourselves as planted instead of buried, and are learning what brings our life into full bloom, the next step is to grow our garden. There are so many ways we can contribute to each other's lives that are essential, insightful, and enlightening—so many ways that we can see each other through the weeds.

Seva stems from two forms of yoga: Bhakti yoga (devotional yoga) and Karma yoga (the yoga of action). Seva is selfless service. It is an act performed without the expectation of selfish reward. Though it can be an act all its own, it can also be an intention folded into those tasks we perform on any given day. Think of ways in which you can give to those around you. Maybe it's as substantial as volunteer work in your community, or assisting someone in need. But when we imbue even our smallest gestures with loving-kindness we can have lasting positive impact on the lives of others. A well-placed compliment or encouragement can provide someone with wind for their sails and the confidence to move forward.

Set an intention. Dedicate your next meditation or yoga practice to something or someone larger than just yourself. That might be a huge worldly cause, but it can also be something more subtle like your friend who is taking the bar exam, your brother who is starting a new job, or your neighbor who's raising three kids on her own. Think of someone or something that could use an extra shot of compassion, and connect with that pure awareness. Notice how it changes how you feel. With a larger purpose in the mix, petty concerns and distractions feel incongruent to the big picture you are plugged into. To quote B. K. S. Iyengar, "It is through your body that you realize you are a spark of divinity."

Just as you are doing with your daily savasanas and your morning and evening meditations, you are going to dedicate at least five minutes every day to **Give Someone Your Attention**. This is you taking the "pay close attention" you're practicing and paying it forward. Your thoughtful awareness is one of the most important gifts you can give, and it is so rewarding on both sides of the equation. Look for opportunities to lift up instead of tear down. When you do, notice how the prejudices you may have held against yourself and others begin to dissolve. Allow yourself to witness that if you are not truly present—not really where you're **at**—attention simply becomes tension like our very first exercise. When we make others feel good, it makes us feel good too—and it motivates us to stay committed to our own "pay close attention" as well. Lest we forget, compassion is defined as "feeling with each other." Of course you can expand on your five minutes any time you want—all I ask is that you **Give Someone Your Attention** consistently without missing a single day.

It's easy to mistake ourselves as separate beings. But all of us are made up of tiny, permeable molecular particles. That means even science and reason suggest that the space inside of us and the space outside of us are one and the same. In Patanjali's Eight-Limbed path, samadhi is the eighth and final fold. It is total immersion and the ultimate stage of yoga. "Sama" (fully integrated, wholeness) and "dhi" (established beyond intellect)—it is to establish the fullest extent of our Supreme consciousness.

Yoga is much more than poses. It's a wonderfully honest friend who isn't afraid to tell us to go back in and change into something better.

It's the yoke of body, mind, and spirit.

And it's our path toward purpose, intelligence, compassion, and love, both within ourselves and toward everything around us.

That's what **OM** is.

**OM** is a capacity we all hold—we just need some encouragement sometimes to get there. We need to remind each other to stay **Close to OM**.

# 16

# Our Ongoing OM

*The end is where we start from.*

—T. S. ELIOT

**YOU'VE COME A LONG WAY FROM** hoisting your sail in our initial savasana and you've reached a place where you can stand aloft and view your progress. Glancing back you see how far you've moved from the harbor—you note the landscape you've left behind and feel the liberation of being at sea. Being at sea has its ups and downs too. But out among the waves you're not anchored or stuck, you're emancipated and ready to S.T.O.P. and S.T.A.R.T., find your balance, and use buoys like your beginner's mind, Val-you, and pratipaksha bhavanam (What's In the Way Is the Way). In this fluid freedom, you never know what the tides might bring, but you can be certain they hold opportunities to use the skillfulness we've cultivated together as you continue to helm your adventure.

Within these pages, you and I have *awakened* to a holistic experience that runs deeper than mere intellectual concepts. We've created an accessible, integrated path from buried

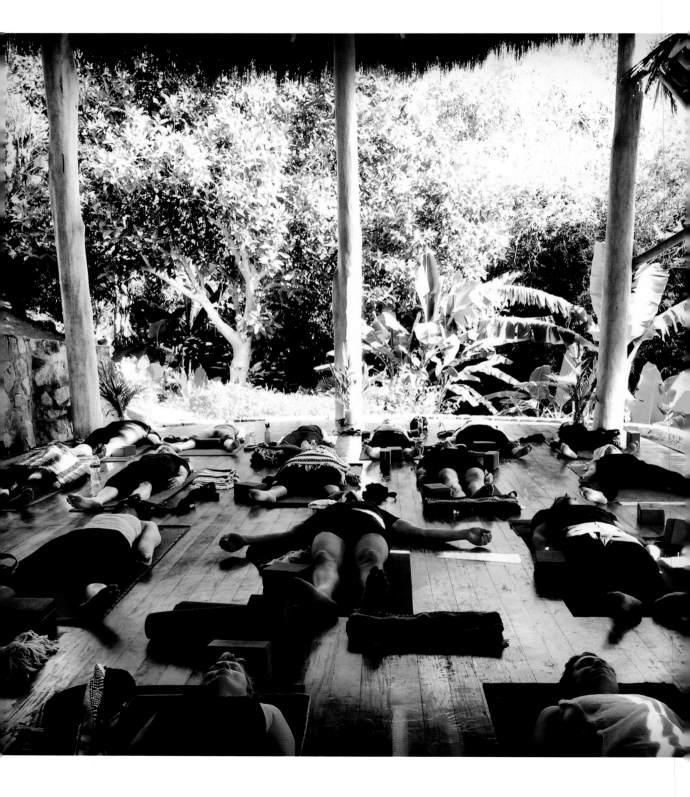

to planted and *transformed* **Stuckat** into a rich personal pilgrimage both on your mat and off. Yoga has *united* us body, mind, and spirit within ourselves and with each other. You might say we've found our **OM**.

**OM** itself is comprised of three sounds: A-U-M. But it is the silence after the last bit of M has faded away that is considered the most expansive and significant. It brings us closest to Ishvarapranidhana:

**Ishvara**—purusha, pure consciousness, creative source

**Pranidhana**—surrender, dedication, practice, devotion

To be **Close to OM** is to live Ishvarapranidhana.

This is not the end of the book but instead the beginning of your new story. As I mentioned earlier, there are no eight-week or twenty-eight-day parameters when it comes to our journey. Ours is truly an ongoing **OM**. I nudged you several times within these pages to ensure that you were clear that you actually have to do this stuff in order for it to work. Well, that's ongoing too.

If you peek ahead, you'll see that you're brushing right up against the appendixes. This is your one-stop-shopping resource for refreshers when it comes to terms, definitions, translations, and deeper explanations for some of the things we touched upon in our chapters. It's also where you'll find sequences of the postures we've done grouped together in various ways that you can use. They'll be written out with illustrations in appendix 1, and audio for them will be available **@OM** as well. In fact, you'll find **Flowing OM**, a single practice that incorporates all the poses we've done in this book. It gives you the arc of a full yoga practice you can access and move through anytime that will bring you **Close to OM** on your mat again and again.

And that's not all. www.closetoOM.com isn't just the home of **@OM**, it's the hub for our community—a place where we can build on our beginner's mind, Val-you, compassion, and learning together. It's a way for us to stay curious and accountable; lose the competition; practice our yoga, meditation, and mindfulness; and live with integrity as part of our ongoing **OM** together. We keep tinkering in our individual laboratories, while enjoying the encouragement of our collective to stay on our path. The interactive blog provides a platform for us to witness each other's stories too. It's our global **Give Some-**

**one Your Attention**. And you'll find regularly updated tips, trips, festivals, and finds, plus information on Seva inspiration and opportunities for us to participate in together.

I look forward to composing our life symphonies together.

And to holding each other **Close to OM**.

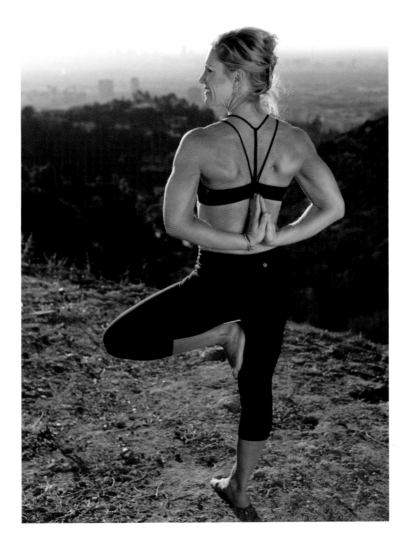

These are short little combinations of postures and sequences we've visited throughout the book grouped together in different ways. Enjoy!

## LET SLEEPING DOGS LIE

5 minute down dog **+** 5 minute savasana.

## CATS AND DOGS

5 rounds of cat/cow **+** 3 minute down dog **+** 5 minute savasana.

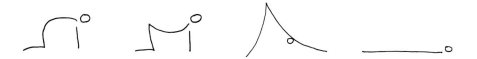

## STEP INTO YOUR MOUNTAIN

3 minutes in tadasana **+** 5 minutes of ABCs **+** 5 minute savasana.

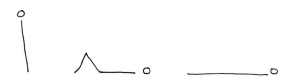

## MOVE MOUNTAINS

1 minutes in tadasana **+** 5 rounds surya namaskar A (pg. 42) **+** 1 minute of ABCs) **+** 5 minute savasana.

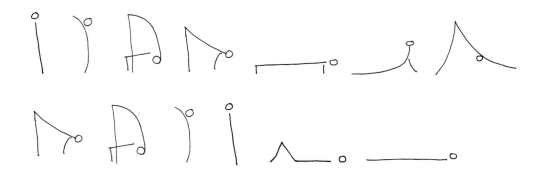

## PEACEFUL WARRIOR

Stand in tadasana facing the long edge of your mat for 1 minute **+** 2.5 minutes in warrior 2, right side (feel free to straighten your leg from time to time to maintain the peace) **+** 5 recovery cycles of breath in tadasana **+** 2.5 minutes in warrior 2 left side **+** 5 cycles of recovery breath in tadasana **+** step back to 1 minute in downward dog or child's pose **+** 1 minute ABCs **+** 5 minute savasana.

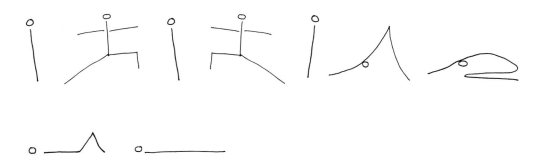

## WITHIN THE REALM OF POSSIBILITY

Begin in child's pose for 1 minute **+** 5 rounds surya namaskar A **+** play with your
Possibility Pose for 5 minutes (you can use crow pose example or any pose you choose)
**+** 1 minute in child's pose **+** 1 minute ABCs **+** 5 minute savasana.

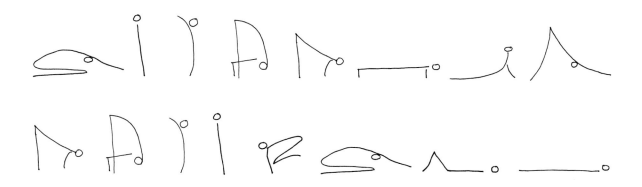

## BUILDING A BRIDGE

1 minute in child's pose **+** 5 rounds surya namaskar A **+** 3 rounds of bridge pose **+**
1 minute of ABCs **+** 5 minute savasana.

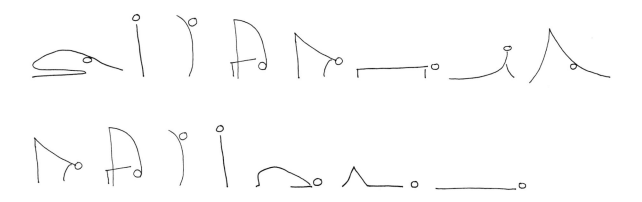

**HARD CORE:** Begin in child's pose for 1 minute **+** 5 rounds surya namaskar A **+** 5 cycles of breath in down dog **+** step from down dog to 2.5 minutes in warrior 2 right side (feel free to straighten your leg if it gets too spicy and find your way back in when you're ready) **+** vinyasa **+** hold down dog for 5 cycles of breath **+** step from down dog to 2.5 minutes in warrior 2 left side **+** step back through a vinyasa or straight into downward dog **+** core work **+** play with your Possibility Pose for 5 minutes (you can use crow pose or any pose you choose) **+** 3 rounds of bridge pose **+** 1 minute ABCs **+** 5 minute savasana.

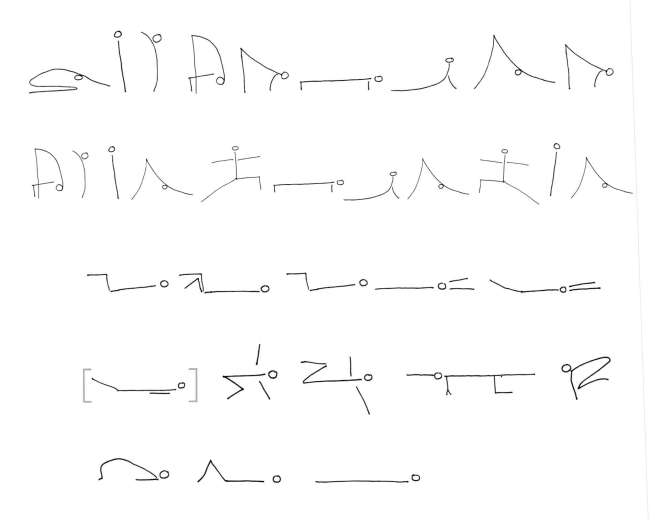

**SOFT CORE**: Core work **+** Possibility Pose **+** 3 rounds of bridge pose **+** 1 minute ABCs **+** 5 minute savasana.

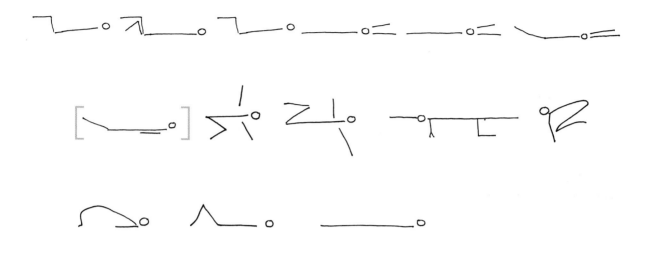

## FOREST FOR THE TREE

**OUT ON A LIMB:** 2 minutes in tadasana **+** tree pose on right side (stay as long as you can balance) **+** 5 cycles of recovery breath in tadasana **+** tree pose on left side (stay as long as you can balance) **+** 5 rounds of surya namaskar A **+** play with your Possibility Pose for 5 minutes (you can use crow pose or any pose you choose) **+** 1 minute ABCs **+** 5 minute savasana.

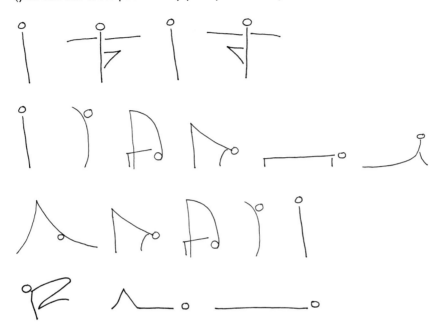

**ROOTS AND BRANCHES:** Begin in child's pose for 1 minute **+** 5 rounds surya namaskar A **+** 1 minute in tadasana **+** tree pose on right side (stay as long as you can balance) **+** 5 cycles of recovery breath in tadasana **+** tree pose on left side (stay as long as you can balance) **+** vinyasa **+** step from down dog to 2.5 minutes in warrior 2 right side (feel free to straighten your leg and find your way back in if the intensity is too rich, just find your way back in when you can) **+** vinyasa **+** 5 rounds of breath in down dog **+** step from down dog to 2.5 minutes in warrior 2 left side **+** step back through a vinyasa or into downward dog **+** core work **+** play with your Possibility Pose for 5 minutes (you can use crow pose or any pose you choose) **+** 3 rounds of bridge pose (some of you who practice *urdhva dhanurasana* might want to add it here) **+** 1 minute ABCs (feel free to place the bottoms of your feet together and let your knees open out to the sides for a gentle hip opener here during your ABCs if you'd like) **+** 5 minute savasana.

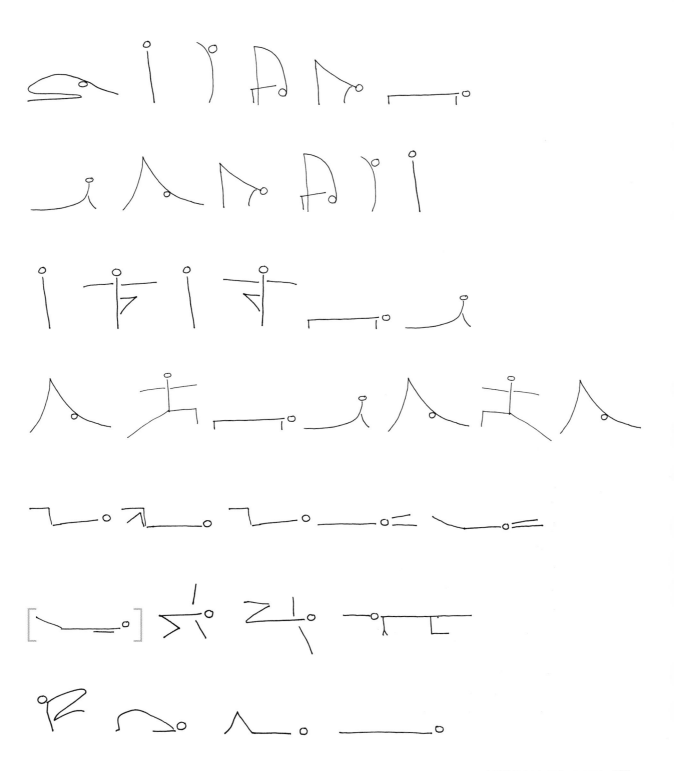

## HEAD TO YOUR HEART

**LIGHTHEARTED**: Begin in child's pose for 1 minute ✚ 5 rounds surya namaskar A ✚ heart-opening sequence including Possibility Pose (you can use crow pose or any pose you choose) ✚ 1 minute ABCs ✚ 5 minute savasana.

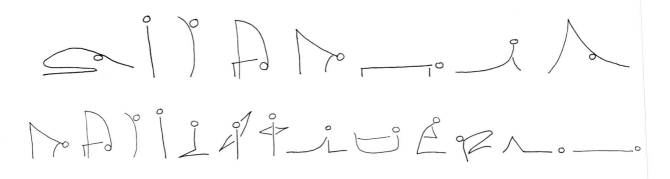

**FULL HEART**: Begin in child's pose for 1 minute ✚ 5 rounds surya namaskar A
✚ 1 minute in tadasana ✚ tree pose on right side (stay as long as you can balance)
✚ 5 cycles of recovery breath in tadasana ✚ tree pose on left side (stay as long as you
can balance) ✚ vinyasa ✚ 5 cycles of breath in down dog ✚ step from down dog to 2.5
minutes in warrior 2 right side (modify by straightening and re-bending the front knee as
needed during this hold) ✚ vinyasa ✚ step from down dog to 2.5 minutes in warrior 2
left side ✚ vinyasa ✚ 5 cycles of breath in downward dog ✚ core work ✚ Possibility Pose
(you can use crow pose or any pose you choose) ✚ heart-opening sequence ✚ 3 rounds
of bridge pose (some of you who practice *urdhva dhanurasana* might want to add it here)
✚ 1 minute ABCs (feel free to place the bottoms of your feet together and let your knees
open out to the side for a gentle hip opener here during your ABCs
if you'd like) ✚ 5 minute savasana.

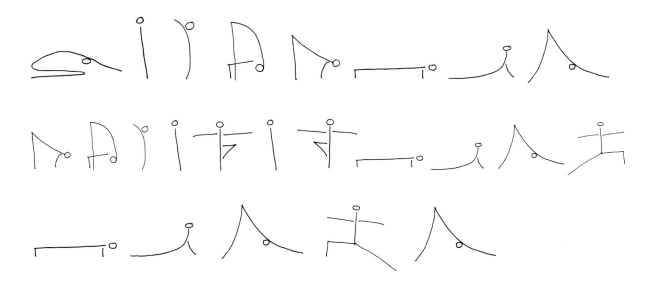

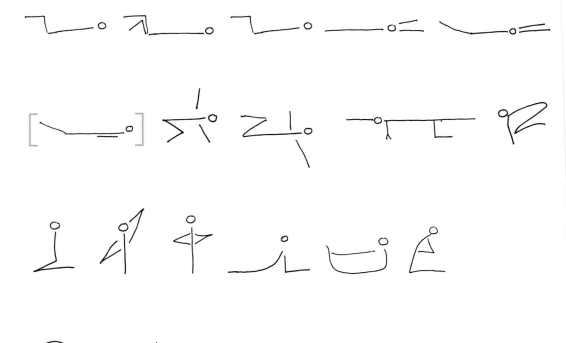

## TWISTS AND TURNS

**A LITTLE BIT TWISTED:** Begin in child's pose for 1 minute **+** 5 rounds surya namaskar A twisting sequence **+** Possibility Pose (you can use crow pose or any pose you choose) **+** heart-opening sequence **+** 3 rounds of bridge pose (some of you who practice *urdhva dhanurasana* might want to add it here) **+** 1 minute ABCs (feel free to place the bottoms of your feet together and let your knees open out to the side for a gentle hip opener here during your ABCs if you'd like) **+** 5 minute savasana.

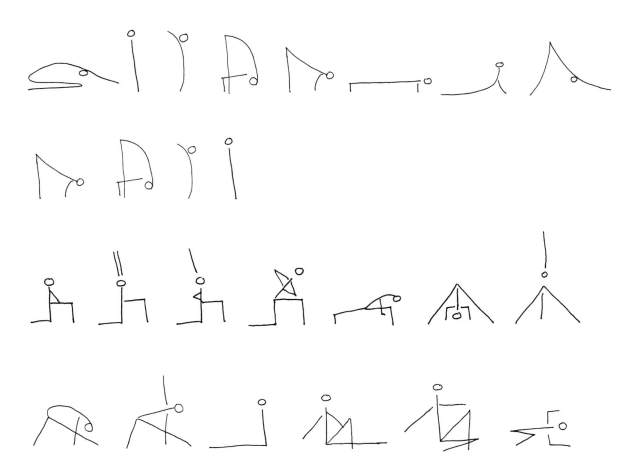

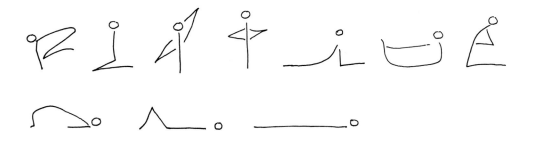

**FULLY TWISTED**: Begin in child's pose for 1 minute ✚ 5 rounds surya namaskar A ✚ 1 minute in tadasana ✚ tree pose on right side (stay as long as you can balance) ✚ 5 cycles of recovery breath in tadasana ✚ tree pose on left side (stay as long as you can balance) ✚ vinyasa ✚ 5 cycles of breath in down dog ✚ step from down dog into 2.5 minutes in warrior 2 right side (modify by straightening and re-bending the front knee as needed during this hold) ✚ vinyasa ✚ step from down dog to 2.5 minutes in warrior 2 left side ✚ vinyasa ✚ 5 cycles of breath in downward dog ✚ core work ✚ Possibility Pose (you can use crow pose or any pose you choose) ✚ twisting sequence ✚ heart-opening sequence ✚ 3 rounds of bridge pose (some of you who practice *urdhva dhanurasana* might want to add it here) ✚ 1 minute ABCs (feel free to place the bottoms of your feet together and let your knees open out to the side for a gentle hip opener here during your ABCs if you'd like) ✚ 5 minute savasana.

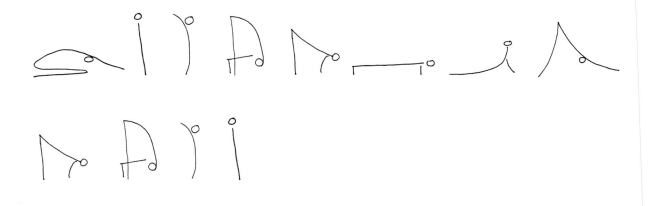

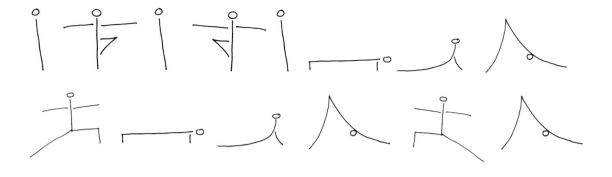

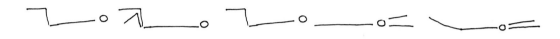

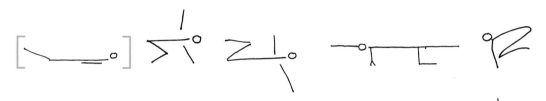

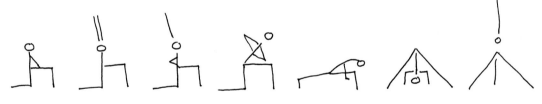

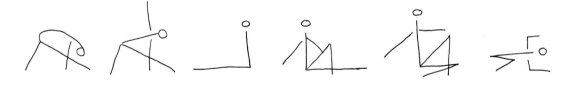

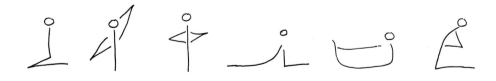

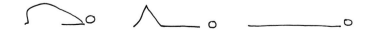

## OM ALONE

Restorative practice and metta meditation **+** 5 minute savasana.

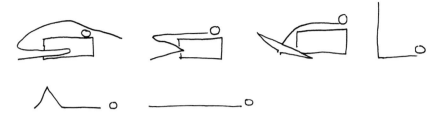

## FLOWING OM

Begin in child's pose for 1 minute **+** 5 rounds surya namaskar A **+** 1 minute in tadasana **+** tree pose on right side (stay as long as you can balance) **+** 5 cycles of recovery breath in tadasana **+** tree pose on left side (stay as long as you can balance) **+** vinyasa **+** 5 cycles of breath in down dog **+** step from down dog into 2.5 minutes in warrior 2 right side (modify by straightening and re-bending the front knee as needed during this hold) **+** straighten the front leg and take triangle pose for 1 full minute **+** vinyasa **+** step from down dog to 2.5 minutes in warrior 2 left side **+** straighten the front leg and take triangle for 1 full minute **+** vinyasa **+** 5 cycles of breath in down dog **+** core work **+** Possibility Pose (you can use crow pose or any pose you choose) **+** twisting sequence **+** heart-opening sequence **+** 3 rounds of bridge pose **+** 1 minute ABCs **+** restorative practice and metta meditation **+** 5 minute savasana.

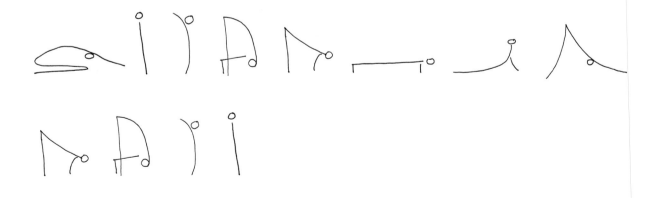

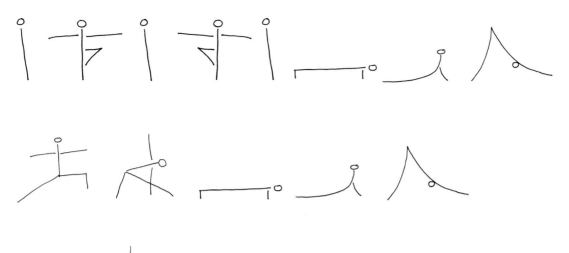

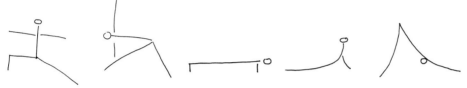

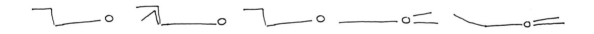

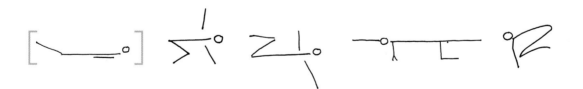

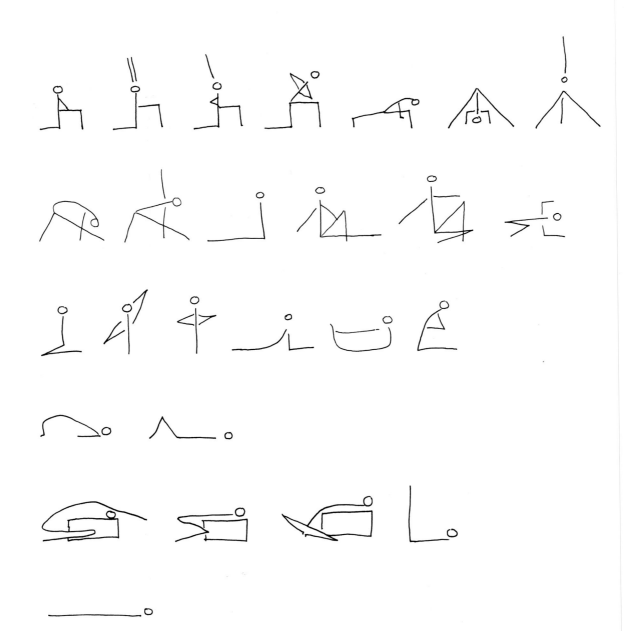

*The Yoga Sutras* was written over 1,700 years ago and contains 195 aphorisms (*sutras* actually means "stitches") of wisdom. They were compiled by a man known as Patanjali, about whom we know very little. *The Yoga Sutras* is a bit of a user's guide for yoga in its larger sense (raja yoga, the "royal" or contemplative aspects of yoga). In fact asanas (the poses) are referenced only a few times within *The Yoga Sutras*. The Eight Limbs (ashtanga) are integrated as a path toward self-realization, spiritual growth, and a purposeful life.

1. **Yamas** Universal moral disciplines.

   *Ahimsa Compassion for all living things.*

   *Satya Truth.*

   *Asteya Non-stealing.*

   *Brahmancharya Control of the senses.*

   *Aparigraha Non-greediness.*

2. **Niyamas** Personal observances.

   *Saucha Cleanliness, clarity, purity.*

   *Santosha A deep-seated sense of contentment.*

   *Tapas Disciplined use of our energy, also defined as "heat."*

   *Svahdyaya Self-study.*

   *Ishvarapranidhana Surrender/dedication to Source, to creative consciousness/God.*

3. **Asana** Yoga postures, comfortable position.

4. **Pranayama** Breath work; life force.

5. **Pratyahara** Withdrawal of the senses.

6. **Dharana** Concentration.

7. **Dhyana** Meditation.

8. **Samadhi** Our true nature, total immersion into pure, unfiltered consciousness.

# GLOSSARY

**ABCs** Awareness, Benevolence, and Calm.

**Abhinivesha** One of the five kleshas associated with "clinging to life."

**Abhyasa** Persevering practice.

**Ahimsa** One of the Eight Limbs, compassion for all living things.

**Alignment** The way in which you align your body in a posture to make it most efficient and beneficial as well as least likely to be injurious.

**Anjaneyasana** A low lunge with your back knee on the ground.

**Aparigraha** One of the yamas in the Eight Limbs. Non-greediness.

**Ardha matsyendrasana** A seated twist.

**Asana** Yoga posture. Comfortable seat.

**Ashtanga** Translates as "eight limbs" and is both a reference to the Eight-Limbed path in Patanjali's *Yoga Sutras* as well as a rigorous style of yoga.

**Asmita** One of the five kleshas associated with ego.

**Asteya** One of the yamas in the Eight Limbs. Non-stealing.

*Yoga Sutras* **Avidya** One of the five kleshas, associated with ignorance.

**Belly Turning (or churning) Pose (jathara parivartanasana)** See instruction and photo on page 97.

**Bhagavad Gita** The Bhagavad Gita is a sacred Hindu scripture and an important historical yogic text written sometime between the fifth and second century BCE.

**Bikram Yoga** A system of twenty-six yoga poses created by Bikram Choudhury and performed in a room heated to 104 degrees F.

**Bound Angle Pose (baddha konasana)** A seated posture with bottoms of the feet together and knees butterflied out to the sides. See the restorative version of this posture (supta baddha konasana) with props on page 172.

**Bow Pose (dhanurasana)** A backbend from your belly. See instruction and photo on page 141.

**Brahmancharya** One of the Eight Limbs. Control of the senses.

**Bridge (setu bandha sarvangasana)** A backbend. See instruction and photo on pages 85–86.

**Camel Pose (ustrasana)** Backbend variation kneeling. See instruction and photo on pages 141–142.

**Cat/Cow (marjaiasana/bitilasana)** Hands and knees posture with movement and breath. See instruction and photo on page 21.

**Child's Pose (balasana)** A resting pose. See instruction and photo on page 47.

**Chitta Vritti** Whirlpools of thought.

**Cobra Pose (bhujangasana)** Part of a sun salutation, cobra is a backbend on your belly and a modified upward facing dog. See instruction and photo on page 47.

**Corpse Pose (savasana)** A relaxation posture lying down on your back, typically visited at the end of a vinyasa flow practice. See instruction and photo on page 16.

**Crow Pose (bakasana)** An intermediate arm balance with knees balancing on the backs of the arms. See photo on page 75.

**Dandasana** Staff pose, seated upright with legs straight out in front of you.

**Dharana** One of the Eight Limbs. Concentration.

**Dharma** "Right" way of living, ultimate path.

**Dolphin Pose (ardha pincha mayurasana)** Down dog on your forearms. See instruction and photo on page 76.

**Downward Dog Pose (adho mukha svanasana)** A pause in every sun salutation that serves as home base. Hands shoulder distance, feet hip distance on the floor, hips high to the sky in a forward folding action. See instruction and photo on pages 27–28.

**Drishti** Concentration Point.

**Dvesha** One of the five kleshas, associated with avoidance.

**Ekagrata** Single pointed focus.

**Gomukhasana** An arm position. See photo on page 138.

**Gunas** Three interdependent qualities of prakriti (nature): Sattva, Rajas, and Tamas.

**Handstand (adho mukha vrksasana)** A posture involving balancing only on your hands. See photo on page 77.

**Hatha** Translates as sun/moon—balance of opposites. It is also an umbrella term for physical practices of yoga, as well as a particular style of postural sequencing.

**Headstand (sirsasana)** Balancing on the top of your head either in a tripod arm variation or with hands interlaced and forearms on the ground.

**Hero's Pose (virasana)** A posture seated between your heels. See instruction and photo on page 104.

**Iyengar** A style of yoga that uses props and emphasizes alignment in postures, created by B. K. S. Iyengar. See boxed material on pages 112–113.

**Koshas** Subtle layers of the Self.

**Kleshas** Five hindrances or obstacles found in Patanjali's *Yoga Sutras*. See pages 148–49.

**Kundalini Yoga** A style of yoga. A synthesis of asana, pranayama (breath work), meditation, and chanting, mantra, and tantra designed to awaken the Kundalini energy and bliss housed in the spine.

**Mantra** "Man" means mind, and "tra" means transport. It's a phrase that's repeated and is often used to drop into meditation.

**Metta** Loving-kindness.

**Midline** A term for the central line, or vertical axis of the body. It is line of energy useful to find balance, stability, and support in postures.

**Modification** Ways in which to adjust postures so that they best suit your body, energy, and experience level. Alternate variations as well as props are fabulous tools to modify your practice so that it feels like the "porridge is just right."

**Namaste** An Indian greeting that translates as "the light in me salutes the light in you." Often spoken at the beginning and/or end of a yoga practice.

**Niyamas** One of the Eight Limbs. Personal observances.

**@OM** Found at www.closetoOM.com for audio and video instruction.

**Prakriti** Nature.

**Pranayama** One of the Eight Limbs. *Prana* translates as "life force" as well as "breath," and *ayama* means restraint. Pranayama is often used as a term for breath work in yoga.

**Prasarita Padottanasana** A wide-legged forward fold with variations. See description and photo on page 156.

**Pratipaksha Bhavanam** What's In the Way Is the Way. The ability to look at a situation from a different perspective and turn negativity into positive action.

**Pratyahara** Inward instead of distractedly outward turn.

**Purusha** Pure consciousness—our highest Self.

**Pyramid Pose (parsvotanansa)** Straight-legged forward fold. See page 156.

**Rajas** One of the three gunas, associated with energy and passion.

**Sadhana** Pilgrimage.

**Samasthiti** Means "even standing" and is another name for tadasana.

**Sama Vritti** Even breathing.

**Samskara** Habits, engrained behavior.

**Sankalpa** Setting an intention with the understanding that we are perfect and whole already, even as we work toward something better.

**Santosha** A deep-seated sense of contentment.

**Sattva** Illumination.

**Satya** Truth.

**Saucha** One of the Eight Limbs. Cleanliness, clarity, purity.

**Shalabhasana** A backbend performed on your belly. See instruction and photo on pages 45–46.

**Single legged crow pose (eka pada bakasana).** See instruction and photo on page 75–76.

**Sphinx (Bhujangasana variation)** Backbend variation on your belly. See instruction and photo on page 140.

**Sthira** Sweetness.

**Stuckat List** A list of those things that make you feel stuck.

**Sukham** Steadiness.

**Supta baddha konasana** A restorative hip-opening posture, which becomes a heart-opener too with props. See instruction on page 172.

**Surya Namaskar A** Sun salutation A. See instruction and photos on page 42. See video of surya namaskar A at closetoOM.com.

**Surya Namaskar B** A sun salutation flow that includes warrior one. See video for surya namaskar b at closetoOM.com.

**Surya Namaskar C** A variation of surya namaskar b. See example at closetoOM.com.

**Svadhyaya** Self-study.

**Tadasana (mountain pose)** See instruction and photo on page 35.

**Tamas** One of the three gunas, associated with inertia.

**Tantra** A style of meditation and ritual that involves using prana (life force energy) to attain spiritual and even mystical liberation. It focuses on the subtle body. Yes, sometimes in relation to sex.

**Tapas** Follow through, discipline, Heat.

**Tree Pose (vrikshasana)** See instruction and photo on page 130–131.

**Triangle Pose (trikonasana)** A straight-legged pose with a wide stance much like warrior 2 but with both legs straight.

**Uddiyana Bandha** Light, lifting engage of the low abdominals. See page 157.

**Ujjayi** Style of breathing used in vinyasa yoga.

**Upvistha Konasana** A wide-legged stretch. See instruction and photo on page 174.

**Upward Facing Dog (urdhva mukha svanasana)** A backbend that is part of vinyasa yoga. See instruction and photo on page 48–49.

**Urdhva Dhanurasana** Full backbend position with hands and feet on the floor and torso arched to the sky. Sometimes called full wheel.

**Urdhva Hastasana** Standing with arms reaching up overhead. See description and photo on page 43.

**Vairagya** Surrender.

**Vajrasana** Seated upon your heels.

**Vinyasa** A style of yoga asana—a series of postures moved by breath—"placed in a deliberate and special way." See descriptions and photos on page 113.

**Viparita Karani** A restorative pose with legs elevated. See instruction and photo on pages 173–74.

**Virasana** Seated between your heels. See instruction and photo on page 104.

**Viveka** Discriminative discernment, aka, the antithesis of impulsive, intoxicated bozos in a bullring.

**Warrior 1 (virabhadrasana 1)** A lunge with your back foot flat on the floor and your torso facing forward, arms shoulder distance overhead. Part of every surya namaskar B. See video for surya namaskar B at closetoOM.com.

**Warrior 2 (virabhadrasana 2)** A standing posture. A lunge in which the torso is open to the side with the arms outstretched. See instruction and photo on pages 59–60.

**Yamas** One of the Eight Limbs. Universal morality.

**Yin Yoga** A style of yoga that moves slowly and holds postures for long periods of time. It's focus is on connective tissue, circulation, and joints as well as inner silence.

**Yoga** Yoke, union, connection. Also refers to physical postures (asanas). See boxed material on page 112.

Baptiste, Baron. *Being of Power*

———. *Journey Into Power*

———. *Perfectly Imperfect: The Art and Soul of Yoga*

Bender Birch, Beryl. *Beyond Power Yoga: 8 Levels of Practice for Body and Soul*

Cope, Steven. *The Wisdom of Yoga: A Seeker's Guide to Extraordinary Living*

———. *The Great Work of Your Life*

Desikachar, T. V. K. *Heart of Yoga*

Easwaran, Eknath. *The Bhagavad Gita for Daily Living, Volume 1: The End of Sorrow*

Farhi, Donna. *Yoga Mind, Body and Spirit: A Return to Wholeness*

Iyengar, B. K. S. *Tree of Yoga*

———. *Light On Yoga*

———. *Light On Life*

Judith, Anodea. *Eastern Body Western Mind*

Kabat-Zinn, Jon. *Everywhere You Go There You Are*

Lasater, Judith Hanson. *Relax and Renew: Restful Yoga for Stressful Times*

———. *Living Your Yoga: Finding the Spiritual in Everyday Life*

Remski, Matthew. *Threads of Yoga: A Remix of Patanjali's Sutras, with Commentary and Reverie*

Salzberg, Sharon. *Real Happiness: The Power of Meditation: A 28-Day Program*

———. http://tricycle.org/magazine/metta-practice/

———. http://www.vipassana.com/meditation/facets_of_metta.php

Singleton, Mark. *Yoga Body: The Origins of Modern Posture Practice*

Warner, Brad. *Hardcore Zen: Punk Rock, Monster Movies and the Truth About Reality*

## FAVORITE MEDIA/PODCAST RESOURCES

Demystifying Patanjali: The Yoga Sutras in Podcasts. https://itunes.apple.com/us/podcast/demystifying-patanjali-the-yoga-sutras/id1038940496?mt=2
On Being: http://www.onbeing.org/tags/yoga
http://www.onbeing.org/program/adele-diamond-the-science-of-attention/transcript/6694
Michael Stone: https://michaelstoneteaching.com/podcasts/
Glorian Publishing: http://gnosticteachings.org/download/practical-spirituality-course.html
Yoga Journal: http://www.yogajournal.com
New York Times: www.nytimes.com/topic/subject/yoga
Kripalu: https://kripalu.org/kripalu-perspectives-podcasts
Insight LA: https://www.insightla.org/audio/guided-meditations
Unplug Meditation: http://unplugmeditation.com/online-classes
MindBodyGreen: http://www.mindbodygreen.com
Mantra Magazine: http://mantramag.com

# ACKNOWLEDGMENTS

When I first started working on the proposal for *Close to OM* with my extraordinary agent, Jane Von Mehren, she slipped me a mantra without even knowing. "This is not a book about you," she told me. I find her words ring true in life as they do in writing, especially when we live into our yoga (#janeismyguru). Then, when Jane introduced me to Daniela Rapp and the entire St. Martin's Press team lay down on the sketchy conference room carpeting for a savasana during our first meeting, I knew I'd found my dream editor and my publishing tribe.

Pat Tobin, I hold you responsible. You encouraged me to write when nobody else noticed. Annie Carpenter, Vinnie Marino, Yogaworks, Michael Edelstein, Jordana Glick-Franzheim, Tamara Taylor, Barbara Menefee Diamond, Christian Donatelli, Liz Hernandez, Julie Pile, Brian Frazer, Sascha Rothchild, Rachel Acheson, and Carissa Eisle: Your input has been invaluable. Sarah Harvison, Jessica Easter, Michelle Greathouse, Kate MacLennan, and my entire lululemon family—your enthusiasm and support are off the charts.

Mama, Eddy, Art, and Dom—I'd have no material without you. Oh, and babe, thank you for understanding that your wife was also married to her manuscript. Emma and Zoe, *the* best kitty-cowriters. Pop, high five up there. We both got our books published the same year! Wish you were here to see it.

I stand in deep, wide gratitude for the incredible teachers and students (some of my most important teachers) who have blessed my path. This is a book about you.

# INDEX

Page numbers in *italics* refer to photographs.